Burning At Both Ends

A Physician's Guide to Surviving Burnout and Reclaiming Purpose in Medicine

Jonathan D. Block, MD, MBA, MLS, MPH, CPE

ISBN — eBook: 979-8-90620-042-6

ISBN — Paperback: 979-8-90620-043-3

ISBN — Hardcover: 979-8-90620-044-0

Disclaimer

This book is intended for informational, educational, and reflective purposes only. It is not medical advice, psychiatric advice, legal advice, financial advice, employment advice, or professional counseling. Nothing in this book creates a physician-patient relationship, attorney-client relationship, financial advisory relationship, coaching relationship, or any other professional relationship between the author and the reader.

The experiences, observations, and recommendations in this book are offered as general guidance for physicians and other clinicians navigating burnout, moral injury, career strain, and professional transition. Readers should use their own judgment and seek qualified medical, mental health, legal, financial, employment, or other professional advice before making decisions affecting their health, licensure, employment, contracts, finances, or clinical practice.

If you are in immediate danger, unable to function safely, or thinking about harming yourself or someone else, seek urgent help immediately through emergency services, a crisis line, a trusted clinician, or another appropriate emergency resource.

Any examples, scenarios, or physician portraits in this book are illustrative. Some may be composites, altered, or fictionalized to protect privacy and confidentiality. Any resemblance to a specific person, practice, institution, employer, insurer, or healthcare organization is coincidental unless otherwise stated.

The author has made reasonable efforts to present accurate and practical information, but healthcare, employment, licensing, financial, and legal environments vary by jurisdiction and change over time. The author and publisher assume no responsibility for errors, omissions, or outcomes resulting from the use or application of the information contained in this book.

Table of Contents

Preface

Burnout has become deeply personal to me, and I never imagined that burnout would be as important as it is. I first encountered physician burnout while serving as department chair at a community teaching hospital. During my tenure, as I transitioned into roles as vice president and president of the medical staff, I formed a committee to address burnout and create a peer support program. A significant challenge is that physicians are often conditioned to be defensive about vulnerability, viewing it as a weakness. Unfortunately, that ingrained isolation creates a lot of unnecessary suffering with often tragic results.

The perfect example of that is something that happened to one of my former partners many years ago. I was working as a private practice urologist in a regional Large Urology Group Practice Association (LUGPA) group. The group had hired a physician to be placed in one of the outlying offices where there was an entrenched and well seasoned Urologist. The financial model at the time created a severe burden on that office, and my partner struggled under the strain of supporting a new hire's salary without company assistance. He never reached out for help, and it is tragic that he saw no other option than to end his life. My wife was very close to him having worked with him routinely, and she was devastated.

Even then, I was oblivious to the burn out in my own life during that situation, though in retrospect, the signs were already showing.

Burnout became more common and prevalent in discussions with my other partners. I remember going into one of my partners' offices one day after scheduled hours were completed to run through a few things and just shoot the breeze. He looked at me directly with a hollow look and said "I don't want to do this anymore." I asked him what he meant to try to pin him down to whether he meant working in the company or doing Urology in general. He looked at me deadpan and said "All of it, I don't want to do any of this anymore, even be in medicine."

That conversation struck me in such a way that I began to realize I, too, was feeling burnout starting a few years ago. I became more and more disgruntled with the system, the burdens of taking call after hours, at night, and on weekends missing functions and events with my family and friends. The burden of after hours work on the electronic medical record taking time every night away from dinner time and socialization with my family was starting to take a real toll. My family and friends began to notice some of the signs before I did where I would become noticeably irritable the nights before having to return to work for the regular work week or even when I was having to do my on call duties the following days. I began to become disgruntled at the requirements and requests from patients. Exacerbating this issue was the corporatization of our practice with the selling to private equity and the new management oversight requirements. The longer I remained in the system, the more pressure was applied.

What is more disconcerting is that I would often mentor and coach others, medical students, residents, colleagues and clients, helping them identify and navigate many of these issues without the self realization that I too was suffering, or at least denying the degree to which I suffered. I would often say medicine was no longer fun to practice.

Collaborating with others in the field eventually opened my eyes to my own burnout. Burnout became personal, and I had to make a hard decision regarding my career. I had wanted to retire early, and fortunately I had set myself in the right positions to be able to do so. I knew I had to pull that trigger for self preservation.

It felt like a huge weight was removed from me when I retired from that practice. I often get asked if the transition was difficult, but the honest answer is that the relief felt far outweighed the trepidation of looking to take on a new role.

Burnout can be understood, survived and even overcome, but only when physicians engage in raw self reflection, brutally honest self-assessment, and the difficult work of naming the truth of what is really happening to them. That is why this book was born.

The Broken Healer: A 2026 Reality Check

The career you trained for is getting shorter.

Medicine hasn't gotten harder to learn. The science hasn't outpaced the clinicians practicing it. The career span is contracting because the system consuming physicians has been optimized for extraction, not sustainability.

Physicians entering practice in 2026 are burning out faster, leaving earlier, and leaving more often than any generation before them. The Permanente 2026 data doesn't leave much room for interpretation: hassle factors, stress trajectories, and early exit rates are all moving in the same direction at the same time. Female physicians are leaving at a median age of 49. Their male counterparts make it to 64. A hazard ratio of 1.43 tells a precise, clinical story about a structural failure that no mindfulness app is going to fix.

You didn't do this.

You survived a training system designed to break you down and rebuild you as something the institution could use. You came out the other side carrying six figures of debt, a schedule someone else controls, a prior authorization queue, and a patient portal full of messages at 10 PM. You kept showing up. The system took that compliance and called it devotion.

This book doesn't call it that.

It calls what's happening what it actually is: a workforce under siege from corporate capture, administrative overload, and a culture that spent decades confusing sacrifice with excellence. And it gives you a practical, unambiguous path out of the siege. Whether that means staying and fighting, shrinking your exposure, moving laterally, or leaving clinical medicine entirely, the decision is yours to make with clear eyes.

Who This Book Is For

You might be the physician who still loves the clinical work but can't sleep on Sunday nights. You might be the one who has run the numbers quietly, trying to figure out if you can actually leave. You might be three years into your first attending job, wondering whether the noncompete clause in your contract means what you think it means.

You might not have said any of this out loud.

This book is for all of those physicians. It's for the one who sat through the last hospital wellness seminar and felt something between rage and exhaustion when the slide deck hit "practice gratitude." It's for the one whose inbox crossed 200 unread messages before noon on a Tuesday. It's for the one who has started running the sunk-cost math on their entire career and doesn't know where to stop.

It's not a book about coping. Coping is what you've already been doing. This is a book about deciding.

How to Use This Manual

Part I diagnoses the injury: what burnout actually is at the biological and psychological level, what moral injury does to a physician over years of blocked care decisions, and why the forces driving early exit can't be absorbed by the individual physician no matter how resilient they are.

Part II names the forces doing the capturing. The private equity playbook. The academic culture that weaponizes the privilege of medicine. The gender attrition data most hospital systems would rather not discuss. The predatory contract clauses that trap physicians before they know the terrain.

Part III is where you start reclaiming agency. It covers tactical boundaries, the mental health and licensure fear that keeps physicians from getting help, financial sovereignty and the Runway Number, and the Four-Path Triage Model that gives you a real decision framework.

Part IV covers the second act: decoupling your identity from the MD credential, building a portfolio career if that's where your triage lands, and following a 12-month operational plan through the transition.

You don't have to read this front to back. If your most pressing problem is a contract you're about to sign, go to Chapter 9. If you're already in crisis, start with Part III. If you need to name what's happening before you can act on it, start here.

A Note on Blame and Responsibility

The system is the problem. That's not a disclaimer. It's a diagnosis. Corporate consolidation, private equity extraction, chronic understaffing, and the administrative machinery of prior authorizations and uncompensated inbox management have created working conditions that wouldn't be tolerated in any other skilled profession.

Holding the system accountable doesn't mean waiting for the system to fix itself. It hasn't fixed itself. It's accelerating.

What this book holds in tension is this: the system caused the injury, and you're the one who has to treat it. That's unfair. It's also true. The pages ahead won't pretend otherwise.

What they will give you is a set of tools, a decision framework, and a clear-eyed account of what your options actually are. The four paths cover the full range: from staying and repairing what's fixable, to building a life outside clinical medicine that uses your intelligence and training in a context that doesn't consume you.

Your degree belongs to you. It always has.

What Burnout Actually Is

The word "burnout" gets used so loosely now that it's lost most of its meaning. A resident pulling a 28-hour shift gets told she's burned out. An attending who snaps at a nurse gets told he's burned out. A physician who finally asks for a lighter panel gets called burned out by her chief in a tone that makes it sound like a character flaw.

None of that is wrong, exactly. But none of it is precise enough to be useful.

Burnout is a specific psychological state. It has a measurable structure. And understanding that structure matters, because the way you diagnose the problem determines what you're actually able to fix. If you think burnout is just fatigue, you'll rest and go back to the same system that broke you. If you think it's an attitude problem, you'll try mindfulness and end up more bitter than before. If you understand what burnout actually is, you can start to see it clearly and make smarter decisions about what to do next.

The Maslach Triad Defined

In the late 1970s, a social psychologist named Christina Maslach started studying human services workers: social workers, nurses, teachers, police officers. She wanted to understand what happened to people who spent their careers dealing with other people's suffering. What she found didn't look like a single symptom. It looked like a syndrome with three distinct dimensions that tended to appear and worsen together.

Maslach called the first dimension emotional exhaustion. This is the depletion that goes deeper than being tired after a long week. It's the feeling that you have nothing left to give at the start of a shift. It's showing up to clinic and realizing, somewhere around 9 AM, that you've already used up whatever you came in with. You can still perform. You can still function. But the internal reserve that used to refill overnight stopped refilling somewhere along the way.

Emotional exhaustion in physicians often gets mistaken for depression or simple overwork. It can look like both. The difference is that it's specifically tied to the giving relationship. You pour out and nothing comes back in. The system keeps drawing from the account while the deposits stop. Over months and years, the balance hits zero.

The second dimension is depersonalization, and this is the one that scares physicians the most when they recognize it in themselves. Maslach described it as developing a detached, callous, or cynical attitude toward the people you serve. In medicine, that means patients start to feel like obstacles, problems to be processed, or sources of more work rather than people who need your help.

Most physicians who reach this point feel enormous shame about it. They became doctors to help people. They chose this career because of some version of genuine care. When they catch themselves resenting a patient for calling the after-hours line, or feeling relief when a procedure gets cancelled, or realizing they don't feel much of anything when they deliver a difficult diagnosis, it doesn't feel like burnout. It feels like becoming a bad person.

It isn't. It's a predictable response to a system that makes genuine human connection structurally impossible. When you have 20 minutes per patient, a chart to document in real time, three pending prior authorizations to fight, and 47 inbox messages waiting after clinic, depersonalization is what the mind does to cope. It's a shield that costs you your humanity and costs patients something real too. But it isn't a character defect. It's a sign that the load has exceeded the structure.

The third dimension is a reduced sense of personal accomplishment. This one is subtle and particularly cruel. Your actual performance may still be solid. Your patients may still have good outcomes. Your colleagues may still respect you. But your internal sense of whether any of it matters has gone quiet.

Physicians talk about this as going through the motions. You do the work but the work doesn't land anymore. You used to feel something when a difficult case resolved well. Now it just means the next case is already waiting. The meaning drain is gradual enough that many physicians don't notice it happening until they realize they can't remember the last time they felt proud of something they did at work.

Together, these three dimensions form what's now known as the Maslach Burnout Inventory framework. Emotional exhaustion, depersonalization, and reduced personal accomplishment. They interact and compound each other. High emotional exhaustion makes depersonalization easier to slip into. Depersonalization produces less satisfying interactions, which erodes the sense of accomplishment. The cycle tightens.

This matters for one practical reason: different dimensions call for different responses. If your primary problem is emotional exhaustion, the answer involves load reduction and recovery time. If your primary problem is depersonalization, you may need structural changes that allow for genuine patient contact again. If the primary driver is the loss of meaning, the intervention looks different still. Treating all three with a meditation app helps nobody.

Institutional Gaslighting

Here's what most healthcare institutions do when their physicians show signs of all three dimensions.

They send an email about a new wellness program. They offer a four-session EAP counseling benefit. They schedule a grand rounds on physician resilience. They remind staff about the gym discount. They post something about mindfulness in the break room.

This is gaslighting. Not accidentally, and not without financial motive.

Gaslighting, at its core, means making someone doubt their own accurate perception of what's happening to them. When a physician correctly identifies that her burnout is caused by a system that assigns her 2,800 patients, pays her on RVU volume, and requires 18 prior authorization clicks per week, and the institution's response is to suggest she hasn't prioritized self-care, the institution is telling her that her accurate read of the situation is wrong. It's her problem. Her coping failure. Her responsibility to fix.

The wellness industry inside medicine has grown enormously over the past decade. Healthcare systems now employ Chief Wellness Officers, run peer support programs, and fund research on physician resilience. Some of that is genuinely useful. But a lot of it serves a different function: it shifts the locus of the problem from the organization to the individual, which protects the institution from having to change anything structural.

If burnout is a resilience deficit, the solution is more resilience training. If burnout is a system design problem, the solution is redesigning the system. The first option costs far less and requires no changes to the revenue model.

The research on this is consistent. Interventions that target individual coping skills alone produce small, short-term improvements that don't hold over time. Interventions that change workload, increase autonomy, improve teamwork, and address workflow problems produce more durable results. The system knows this. The system continues to invest heavily in the former.

When you participate in your institution's wellness program and still feel terrible six months later, the unspoken message from leadership is that you didn't try hard enough or want it badly enough. This is the gaslighting loop. You did the thing they prescribed. The thing didn't work. The failure gets attributed to you.

Naming this clearly doesn't mean therapy is useless or that individual coping has no role. It means that framing systemic injury as a personal failure serves the institution and harms the physician. Once you see that framing for what it is, you can stop measuring yourself against it.

Moral Distress vs. Burnout: A Critical Distinction

Burnout and moral distress are related, and in clinical medicine they often occur together. But they're different enough that confusing them leads to wrong interventions.

Burnout, as Maslach defined it, is fundamentally about chronic occupational stress. It's what happens when the demands of the job consistently exceed your capacity to meet them over a long period of time. The cause is volume, pace, overload, and depletion. It doesn't require a specific values conflict. A financial analyst can burn out. A teacher can burn out. Burnout happens across industries and professions whenever people are chronically overextended.

Moral distress is something more specific. It describes the psychological weight of knowing what the right course of action is, and being prevented from taking it. The concept was first developed in nursing literature and has since been applied to physicians with considerable force, because medicine puts doctors in this position constantly.

You know a patient needs a medication. The prior authorization is denied. You appeal. It gets denied again. The patient goes without. You did everything the system allows and the right thing still didn't happen.

You know a patient should be admitted. The bed manager tells you there are no beds. You send the patient home knowing they'll be back in 24 hours, possibly worse.

You know the correct procedure, but your productivity metrics require you to see another patient in the next 18 minutes.

In every one of these situations, the problem isn't exhaustion. The problem is that you've been made complicit in something that violates your professional values, and the system made you complicit while telling you it was your job to be okay with it.

Moral distress accumulates. Physicians who carry it long enough develop what some researchers call moral residue, the lingering weight of decisions where they compromised what they believed was right. Over time, moral distress can feed into all three Maslach dimensions. It accelerates emotional exhaustion, triggers depersonalization as a protective response, and devastates the sense of accomplishment because you're no longer measuring accomplishment against "did I do good medicine?" but against "did I get through the day?"

The distinction matters because the coping strategies are different. Burnout responds to load reduction and recovery. Moral distress responds to restoring the physician's ability to act in alignment with their values, either by changing the constraints or by changing the environment entirely.

Many physicians who describe themselves as burned out are actually describing a combination of both. The exhaustion is real. So is the moral injury. The wellness program addresses neither.

Chapter 2 goes deeper into moral injury and how the prior authorization system turned it into a daily event. For now, the key distinction to hold is this: exhaustion and values violation are both real, they often co-occur, and they need different responses.

The Prevalence Data

Physician burnout rates have been measured across specialties, settings, and career stages for roughly two decades. The consistent finding across major surveys is that more than half of practicing physicians report at least one symptom of burnout at any given time. Some surveys, depending on how they define burnout and which population they sample, find rates significantly higher.

The data isn't clean. Different studies use different measurement tools. The Maslach Burnout Inventory, the Mini-Z, and various single-item screening questions don't always agree with each other. And burnout fluctuates. A physician who scores high in March during flu season and performs well in August after vacation may show up differently in different survey windows.

But even with measurement limitations, the pattern holds across decades and across countries. Physicians in the United States report burnout at rates that would be treated as a crisis in any other industry. Emergency medicine, internal medicine, family medicine, and OB/GYN consistently appear among the highest-burnout specialties. Surgeons and proceduralists report high rates too, often concentrated in different Maslach dimensions.

What's changed most sharply in recent years isn't the overall burnout rate, which has been high for a long time. It's the intention to leave. Surveys tracking physician career intentions show a meaningful increase in the proportion of physicians who are actively considering reducing their clinical hours, leaving their current employer, or leaving clinical medicine entirely within the next two years. The burnout rate was already elevated before the COVID-19 pandemic. The pandemic didn't create the problem; it accelerated it and made its consequences more visible.

The physician workforce math on this is stark. The United States was already projected to face a physician shortage over the next decade, driven largely by an aging population needing more care and an aging physician workforce retiring. When you add accelerated burnout-driven attrition to that equation, the shortage projections get worse. And when experienced physicians leave, they take years of clinical judgment, subspecialty knowledge, and mentorship capacity with them.

This isn't background noise. It's the operating environment you're working in right now.

One more prevalence finding worth sitting with: burnout doesn't fall evenly across the physician population. Women physicians report higher rates than men across most studies. Physicians in employed settings, which now describes the majority of practicing physicians in the United States, report higher rates than those in independent practice. Physicians early in their careers report high rates, driven partly by student debt and loan-driven practice decisions. Physicians in the middle of their careers report high rates, driven partly by the accumulated weight of years in a system that doesn't change. And physicians in the final third of their careers report high rates, driven partly by watching the profession they trained for become something they don't recognize.

The variance matters because it tells you where the system pressure is concentrated. It's not random. It clusters around the features of the modern physician experience that have changed most dramatically in the last two decades: the shift to employment, the administrative load, the loss of autonomy, and the erosion of the patient relationship.

What This Means for You Right Now

Knowing the framework doesn't fix anything by itself. But it does two important things.

First, it gives you language. When you can name emotional exhaustion as distinct from depersonalization as distinct from loss of meaning, you can start to identify which dimension is hitting you hardest. That changes what you look for, what you try to change, and what you ask for. A physician who is primarily exhausted needs different things than a physician who is primarily experiencing the loss of meaning from moral distress.

Second, it removes the self-blame frame. Burnout is not a failure of grit. Depersonalization is not a character flaw. Leaving clinical medicine is not giving up. These are predictable responses to a system that was designed for production, not for physicians, and certainly not for patients.

Your institution may continue to send wellness emails. Your chief may continue to suggest you try better time management. Your department may run another survey, see the same results, and schedule another Grand Rounds on resilience.

You don't have to accept the framing that puts the problem in your hands when the problem lives in the structure.

The chapters ahead map out what the structure actually looks like, how it was built, who benefits from it, and what you can do about it. That starts with understanding the specific mechanics of the system that keeps physicians in a state of managed exhaustion, which is where the next chapter begins.

For now, three things worth doing:

Pull out the Maslach Burnout Inventory and score yourself honestly. It's publicly available and takes about ten minutes. Look at your scores across all three dimensions, not just the overall picture. Notice which dimension is highest. Write it down.

Identify one thing in your current work environment that you believe is a structural problem, not a personal coping failure. Name it specifically: not "I'm overwhelmed" but "I have 23 minutes per patient and documentation takes 12 of them." Concrete language about concrete constraints is more actionable than vague distress.

Notice the next time your institution's response to a systemic problem is a program aimed at individual resilience. You don't have to say anything. Just notice it. The pattern becomes easier to see once you know what you're looking for.

Moral Injury and the Permission Slip Economy

There's a specific kind of exhaustion that comes from knowing exactly what your patient needs and being blocked from providing it. You have the training. The evidence supports the decision. But someone at an insurance company, often with no medical background, decided the answer is no.

That experience is moral injury. It's worth distinguishing from burnout, because the two require different responses and the difference changes what you do next.

Defining Moral Injury in Clinical Medicine

The term moral injury comes from military medicine. Psychiatrist Jonathan Shay used it to describe what happens when soldiers are ordered to act against their moral code, or when they witness something that violates it. The wound isn't grief in the ordinary sense. It's the damage done when you betray what you believe is right, or when a system forces your hand in that direction.

Medicine borrowed the term for good reason.

When a physician is trained to put the patient first, and then placed inside a system that routinely makes that impossible, something breaks. Burnout is depletion. Moral injury is corruption. Burnout says "I'm empty." Moral injury says "I'm complicit in something wrong."

This distinction matters because the standard response to burnout, workload reduction, schedule restructuring, restored autonomy, doesn't fully touch moral injury. You can shorten your clinic day and still carry the weight of every patient you couldn't help, every treatment you couldn't deliver, every time the system overruled you.

Moral injury requires something else first: naming what happened. Saying clearly that a system routinely blocking medically necessary care for financial reasons is doing something wrong, and your distress about it is an appropriate response.

The medical culture has historically treated that distress as a coping failure. The resilience lectures, the wellness committees, the suggestion that you need better stress management skills. All of it assumes the physician's response is the variable needing adjustment, not the situation causing it.

That framing is gaslighting. The rest of this chapter explains why.

The Prior Authorization Machine

Prior authorization was designed as a cost-control tool. The idea was that insurers would review certain high-cost treatments before approving them, catch unnecessary utilization, and save money. That was the pitch.

In practice, it became something else entirely.

According to AMA 2026 data, 44% of physicians report being unable to deliver care they deemed medically necessary because of prior authorization denials. Nearly half. That means almost one in two physicians is regularly stopped from doing their job by an administrative process that has nothing to do with clinical judgment.

That number deserves a moment. This isn't physicians being blocked from experimental treatments or fringe therapies. This is standard-of-care medicine. MRIs. Specialist referrals. Medications that have been first-line for years. Denied.

The typical prior authorization process involves submitting clinical documentation, waiting for a decision, appealing if denied, waiting again, sometimes requesting a peer-to-peer review, and waiting again. Each step burns physician time. Each step delays patient care.

What makes this particularly corrosive isn't only the time cost. It's that you know what needs to happen. Your patient knows what needs to happen. And you're both sitting there while a process designed by actuaries, managed by health plan employees who may never have treated a patient, tells you both to wait.

The peer-to-peer review is where the moral injury becomes most visible. You, a trained physician, have to call and argue your clinical case to a physician employed by the insurer. Sometimes that reviewer is in your specialty. Often they're not. You lay out the evidence, the guidelines, the patient's specific situation. And then they say no anyway.

Most physicians describe this as one of the most demoralizing experiences in modern practice. The conversation isn't clinically valuable. The insurer's reviewer isn't offering a second clinical opinion based on an independent assessment. The whole exchange exists to slow you down enough that some patients give up and some physicians stop appealing.

It's a delay tactic with a medical veneer.

The Permission Slip Economy

The phrase "permission slip economy" captures what medicine has quietly become. A permission slip economy is one where the physician's clinical authority has been systematically subordinated to a layer of administrative approval. You can diagnose. You can recommend. You can write the order. But you can't deliver without permission.

This didn't happen in a single policy change. It was constructed gradually through contracts, insurance plan design, EMR workflows, and the slow normalization of prior auth as just part of the job. Each individual step seemed manageable. The cumulative effect is that physicians now operate inside a system where their clinical judgment is technically respected but practically overruled on a daily basis.

Think about what that does to professional identity. You spent four years in medical school and three to seven years in residency developing clinical judgment that extracted an enormous personal toll. You trained to make decisions about patient care.

Now a substantial portion of your workday is spent justifying those decisions to people who aren't clinicians, or navigating systems designed to say no first.

The permission slip economy has a second layer that's less discussed. It's not just that you need approval to treat patients. The whole culture of modern healthcare has been built around the assumption that physicians need to be checked. Quality metrics. Audit systems. Documentation requirements. Productivity benchmarks. Patient satisfaction scores. Each mechanism carries an implicit message: your judgment alone isn't enough.

Some accountability structures serve real purposes. Documentation matters. Quality data matters. But the current system has gone far past accountability into surveillance. When you're spending hours every week documenting not because it helps the patient but because it protects the institution legally and satisfies payer requirements, something has shifted.

Survey data is consistent across sources: loss of autonomy ranks among the top drivers of physician burnout. Physicians report it ahead of compensation, ahead of call burden, ahead of workload in the abstract. The feeling that their expertise counts. When you systematically remove that, you don't get a more efficient physician. You get a burned-out one.

When Saying No to Patients Is Part of the Job Description

One of the most underdiscussed consequences of the permission slip economy is what it demands emotionally from physicians.

You're the one in the room with the patient. You ordered the test they need. You wrote the prescription for the medication that works. And now you have to explain why they can't have it yet, or why the insurance company denied it, or why you need to try a cheaper drug first that you know is less effective for this specific person.

This is called "step therapy" or "fail first" protocols. They require patients to try and fail on a lower-cost treatment before the insurer will approve what you actually prescribed. In some cases, the required treatment can cause harm. In others, it delays effective care by weeks or months.

You know this. Your patient is looking at you. And you have to say we have to try this other option first because the insurance company requires it.

Every one of those conversations is a small fracture. You're communicating something that contradicts what you believe is true. You're not lying. But you're delivering the insurer's financial decision as though it's a clinical reality.

Multiply that by the number of patients you see in a week. Multiply it by months, then years. The weight is cumulative.

Physicians don't talk about this enough in formal settings because the system has normalized it. Prior auth is just part of practice now. It's expected. But normalization doesn't mean it's not damaging. It means the damage has become invisible.

The Moral Math of Prior Authorization

Consider what 44% looks like in a working week.

If you see 20 patients in a day, and nearly half of them need something you can't immediately deliver because of prior authorization, that's roughly 8 to 10 patients leaving your office without the care they need today. Maybe they'll get it next week. Maybe they'll give up and not appeal. Maybe they'll land in the emergency department with a worsening condition that could have been managed in your office.

Each of those outcomes represents a clinical failure that you were powerless to prevent.

AMA surveys have consistently found physicians spending more than a full workday every week on prior authorization tasks: clinical documentation, peer-to-peer reviews, appeals, and the decision-making underneath all of it. That's time that isn't spent on patient care. On education. On anything that restores the physician rather than depleting them.

That time is also uncompensated. You don't bill for prior auth work. Your RVU count doesn't reflect it. Your employer's productivity metrics don't capture it. It's absorbed into the professional expectation that physicians will do whatever it takes.

That phrase has been weaponized against doctors for decades. It's the implicit justification for every unpaid hour, every border crossed, every burden added. You chose medicine. You took an oath. Whatever it takes.

The oath was to the patient. It wasn't to the insurer's denial workflow.

Moral Injury vs. Burnout: Why the Difference Changes What You Do Next

Chapter 1 defined burnout through the Maslach framework: exhaustion, cynicism, and reduced efficacy. Moral injury sits in different territory.

Burnout can develop in any high-demand, low-control environment. It's a human response to chronic overload without adequate recovery. It doesn't require a values betrayal, just a sustained imbalance between demand and resource.

Moral injury is specific. It requires that something you believe is right gets compromised, either by your own action or by a system that forces your hand. In clinical medicine, the most common mechanism is exactly what we've been describing: you know what's right for your patient, and the system won't let you deliver it.

Recovering from moral injury requires naming what happened. Saying clearly: a system that denies medically necessary care for financial reasons is doing something wrong, and my distress about it is appropriate. That distress is signal. A well-calibrated one.

Burnout often responds to workload reduction and restored autonomy. Moral injury doesn't fully resolve with those things, because the wound is ethical. You can reduce your patient panel and still carry the weight of every prior auth denial that delayed care, every peer-to-peer you lost, every patient who fell through the gap.

The healing starts not with a schedule change but with permission to stop calling your reaction a personal failing.

The Cumulative Toll

Moral injury doesn't arrive as a single breaking point for most physicians. It accumulates.

It's the prior auth denial that delayed a patient's cancer workup by three weeks. It's the step therapy requirement that forced a patient to fail on a cheaper antidepressant before you could prescribe what you knew they needed. It's the peer-to-peer call where you explained the clinical rationale for 20 minutes and received a no in four words.

It's the patient who cried in your office because they can't afford the out-of-pocket cost of the approved alternative, and all you can do is search for samples or discount cards while your next patient waits.

Each incident feels manageable in isolation. You push through it. You move to the next patient, finish the clinic day. But these incidents don't fully clear. They stack.

Research on moral injury in other high-stakes professions shows that accumulation works differently than acute events. A single terrible day can shake a person, but humans are built to recover from acute events. Chronic, repeated exposure to situations where you can't do the right thing is more corrosive because it reshapes expectations. You stop being surprised by the denial. You start anticipating it. You begin calibrating your clinical decisions not by evidence alone but by what the insurer will likely approve.

That's the part nobody discusses in grand rounds.

When you start making clinical decisions with one eye on the prior auth process, your autonomy isn't just impaired from the outside. The constraint has been absorbed into your thinking. You've internalized it.

This is the deepest mechanism of the permission slip economy. Outright denial of care is visible. The way denials reshape physician thinking over time is nearly invisible.

The Systems That Benefit From Silence

Prior authorization denials are profitable.

This is not a conspiracy. It's a straightforward financial calculation. Every day a denial delays a procedure, a medication, or a specialist visit is a day the insurer holds on to that premium dollar. A percentage of patients don't appeal. A percentage of physicians don't have time to fight every denial. Approval rates go up on resubmission, but only for the cases where someone had the bandwidth to push back.

The system is designed to create friction. And friction, in this context, has a dollar value.

Understanding this doesn't make the individual physician feel better on a Tuesday afternoon when they're on hold for a peer-to-peer call. But it matters for how you frame what's happening to you. You're not struggling to cope with an inefficient system that no one has gotten around to fixing. You're pushing against a system that works exactly as designed, and whose design does not center your patient's care.

That's a different diagnosis, and it calls for a different response.

The healthcare advocacy space has made progress. Several states have enacted prior authorization reform laws requiring faster turnaround times and limiting step therapy in certain contexts. Gold carding, where physicians with strong approval track records are exempted from routine prior auth review, has gained traction in some markets. These are real wins, even if they're slow and insufficient on their own. The fact that reform is possible confirms that the current system is a policy choice, not a permanent feature of medical practice.

What You Can Do Right Now

Knowing the mechanism behind moral injury matters. And this book is a manual, so here's what's actionable today.

Track your prior auth burden. Start logging the number of prior auth requests your practice submits each week, the denial rate, and your approximate time cost. Not for institutional reporting purposes. For yourself. When you see the hours accumulate in writing, it reframes your situation from vague exhaustion into a concrete, measurable problem. It also becomes useful data if you ever negotiate your contract or make a case to an employer about administrative overhead.

Separate your clinical judgment from the administrative record. When you document a peer-to-peer or an appeal, include your clinical rationale fully and clearly. Your reasoning should be legible even when the system ignores it. This protects the patient and creates a paper trail of your professional judgment that exists independently of the insurer's decision.

Know your state's prior authorization laws. Many states now require insurers to respond to urgent prior auth requests within 24 to 72 hours. Some have enacted gold carding provisions. Some prohibit step therapy in specific drug classes. Knowing what the law requires in your state gives your staff concrete grounds for escalation and lets you hold insurers to timelines they're legally obligated to meet.

Appeal every time the clinical picture warrants it. Denial rates drop sharply at first appeal. The system counts on a percentage of physicians not having time to fight. Be the one who does, when the clinical evidence genuinely supports it. You won't win every time. But consistent appeal behavior shifts the insurer's calculation and creates a record of the care you tried to deliver.

Talk to your peers about this. The isolation of moral injury is part of its weight. Physicians who talk to each other about these experiences consistently find that their distress is a shared response to a shared problem. Specialty societies, local medical staff organizations, and informal peer networks all serve this function. The recognition that you're not uniquely struggling to cope does something that a wellness lecture can't.

The prior auth machine won't be dismantled this week. The permission slip economy won't disappear because you named it. But naming it clearly changes how much power it holds over your professional identity. You're not failing to cope. You're a trained physician responding appropriately to a system that routinely asks you to act against your clinical values.

That response is information. And the rest of this book is about what to do with it.

The System Pathology

The research doesn't start with a dramatic headline. It starts with a question someone finally decided to ask: what are the specific, day-to-day hassles that are grinding physicians down? Not burnout as an abstraction. Not "physician wellness" as a talking point. The actual, granular, identifiable friction points that stack hour after hour until a good doctor starts calculating how many years are left before escape becomes possible.

That's the frame of the Permanente 2026 research on hassle factors, stress, and early exit trajectories. And when you see the categories laid out, what hits you isn't shock. It's recognition. The data maps what physicians already know in their bones but have been told to stop naming out loud.

The system is sick. The physicians working inside it are showing the symptoms. And every time leadership hands out a mindfulness handout or announces a new wellness initiative, they're treating the patient with a bandage while the hemorrhage continues underneath.

The Permanente 2026 Data

Permanente researchers didn't set out to prove that physicians are unhappy. They set out to understand the specific mechanisms driving stress and early exit, because those mechanisms have a direct line to physician supply, patient access, and long-term system viability. The research identified hassle factors as a primary category of occupational stress, distinct from the emotional weight of clinical work itself.

Hassle factors are the non-clinical demands layered on top of clinical care. They're the administrative overhead, the documentation friction, the scheduling complexity, the approval loops, and the bureaucratic processes that consume physician time without producing patient value. The Permanente data confirmed what many physicians already suspected: it's not the medicine that's breaking people. It's everything surrounding the medicine.

That's a critical distinction. The physicians who entered medicine understood that it would be hard. They accepted the long hours in training, the emotional weight of patient care, the years of deferred income. What they didn't sign up for was spending a substantial portion of their working lives on tasks that have nothing to do with patient care and that, in many cases, actively interfere with it.

The research connected hassle factor burden directly to stress levels, and stress levels directly to early exit intention. The trajectory isn't random. Physicians who reported high hassle factor loads were significantly more likely to report serious consideration of leaving clinical medicine ahead of traditional retirement age. The pipeline isn't just leaking at the top because of burnout. It's leaking across career stages because the daily friction has become unsustainable.

What makes this data powerful is that it reframes the exit conversation. Physicians who leave early often get labeled as "not cut out for it," as if the problem is personal fitness for a demanding profession. The Permanente research says something different: the problem is measurable system dysfunction, and the physicians leaving are responding rationally to an irrational environment.

The data also matters because it gives physicians language. When you can point to a documented research framework that names your experience as a structural problem, you stop internalizing it as a personal failure. That reframe is the first step toward making a clear-headed decision about what to do next.

Mapping the Pressure Points

Hassle factors don't arrive as one large, obvious injury. They accumulate as dozens of small frictions, each one manageable on its own, that compound into something genuinely damaging over time. To understand the system pathology, you have to map these pressure points specifically.

Documentation burden sits at the center of the stack. The EHR was sold to medicine as an efficiency tool. In practice, for most physicians, it functions as an administrative tax on every patient encounter. The time required to document a visit often rivals or exceeds the time spent with the patient. That's not a technology problem in isolation. It's a policy and incentive problem. Insurers, regulators, and liability standards all demand documentation at a level that has nothing to do with clinical care quality and everything to do with billing capture and legal protection. The physician is the one bearing the cost.

Scheduling complexity is the second major pressure point. Patient panels have expanded. Visit windows have compressed. The math on this is simple: more patients in less time means less time per patient, which means more cognitive rushing, more clinical compromise, and more end-of-day charting to cover what couldn't get done during the visit. Administrators who have never seen a patient in a clinical setting often set these schedules based on throughput metrics rather than clinical reality.

Approval and authorization loops were covered in detail in Chapter 2, but it's worth naming them here as a hassle factor in their own right, separate from the moral injury angle. Even when a physician isn't experiencing the full moral weight of a denied authorization, the sheer time cost of navigating those loops is a legitimate work burden. Every prior authorization request is uncompensated administrative labor. Multiplied across a week, a month, a career, it adds up to thousands of hours.

Meeting proliferation is a quieter pressure point but a real one. The corporate capture of medical institutions has brought with it the corporate meeting culture. Committee meetings, quality metric reviews, compliance trainings, departmental town halls, "physician engagement" sessions. Many of these have no discernible effect on patient care. They do have a discernible effect on physician schedules, which are already stretched beyond reasonable limits.

Inbox and message load will get its full treatment in Chapter 4, but it belongs in this map. The portal message queue, the internal communication platforms, the after-hours paging, the results that need review, the referrals that need coordination. All of it lands in a physician's lap outside of scheduled clinical time, largely uncompensated, largely expected.

Autonomy erosion runs through all of these pressure points as a common thread. When a physician can't control their schedule, can't make clinical decisions without administrative approval, can't manage their inbox volume, and can't push back on committee assignments without social or professional consequences, what they've lost is agency. And the loss of agency is corrosive in a way that raw workload alone is not. People can sustain heavy workloads when they feel control over their work. They can't sustain moderate workloads when they feel completely at the mercy of a system that doesn't respect their judgment.

The cumulative picture these pressure points create is not a collection of inconveniences. It's a structural argument that the modern physician's job has been redesigned, piece by piece, away from the clinical work physicians are trained and motivated to do, toward an administrative and compliance function that serves institutional and payer interests instead.

Why Individual Resilience Cannot Fix a Structural Problem

At some point in the last decade, someone decided that the correct response to this structural problem was to help physicians become more resilient. More mindful. Better at self-care. The wellness industry inside healthcare grew into a significant enterprise, offering meditation apps, resilience workshops, peer support groups, and "physician wellness champions" whose job was to help their colleagues cope.

None of this is inherently wrong. Taking care of yourself matters. Having social support matters. But when these offerings are presented as the solution to the system pathology mapped above, they cross from supportive to insulting.

Here's the problem with resilience as a primary intervention: it assumes the issue is inadequate individual coping. It locates the dysfunction inside the physician rather than inside the system. And that mislocation is not accidental. It's far cheaper to run a mindfulness workshop than to fix scheduling ratios, reduce documentation burden, eliminate unnecessary committees, or restructure compensation models. Resilience programming shifts the cost of system dysfunction from the institution onto the physician.

Research on occupational health has consistently shown that sustainable work requires not just individual resources but structural conditions: reasonable workload, clear expectations, adequate control over one's work, fair treatment, a sense of community, and alignment between personal and organizational values. When the structural conditions are broken, individual coping strategies become a holding action, not a solution. You can only hold so long before the structure wins.

The math on this is also straightforward. If a physician's job generates more stress than any reasonable coping strategy can absorb, adding more coping strategies doesn't fix the deficit. It just delays the moment of collapse. The Permanente 2026 data on early exit trajectories reflects exactly this dynamic. Physicians aren't leaving because they ran out of resilience. They're leaving because they correctly assessed that no amount of individual adaptation would change the structural conditions they were working within.

The wellness lecture circuit does something even more damaging than offering an inadequate solution. It implies that physicians who are struggling have a personal deficiency. The message, underneath the supportive language, is: "Your colleagues are managing fine. If you're burning out, you need to work on yourself." That message is a lie, and it lands on top of an already heavy professional culture of stoicism and shame. Chapter 12 will cover the shame machine in detail. For now, recognize that any institution that responds to a structural problem with individual wellness programming is engaged in a form of gaslighting, whether leadership intends it that way or not.

The structural problem needs a structural analysis. That's what this chapter is providing. And structural analysis is the precondition for structural action, which is what the rest of this book is about.

The Organizational Diagnosis

If a physician presented to clinic with the symptoms the healthcare system is displaying, the workup would lead to a clear diagnosis. The organizational body is sick, and the sickness has identifiable features.

Incentive misalignment is the first and most central finding. The dominant business model of corporate healthcare prioritizes volume, billing capture, and short-term margin. Physician wellbeing, clinical quality, and long-term workforce sustainability are secondary concerns when they appear on the balance sheet at all. When the financial incentives of an institution point in a different direction than the clinical values of its physicians, conflict is the predictable result. Physicians feel it as moral distress. Administrators call it a communication problem. Both framings are wrong about the cause.

The incentive misalignment isn't a personality clash between caring physicians and uncaring administrators. Most administrators aren't villains. They're operating inside their own set of pressures: investor expectations, board mandates, regulatory compliance, margin targets, and market competition. The problem is that those pressures systematically de-prioritize the conditions under which physicians can do their best work. The result is a structural collision that produces predictable damage at the physician level.

Administrative bloat is the second diagnostic finding. The ratio of administrative to clinical staff in U.S. healthcare institutions has shifted dramatically over the past two decades. More administrators, more compliance officers, more quality metric managers, more prior authorization staff, and more billing coders share overhead with a physician workforce whose numbers haven't kept pace. Every additional administrative layer generates additional demands on physician time through documentation requirements, meetings, sign-offs, and approvals. The physician at the center of this structure isn't being supported by it. They're being administered by it.

Disconnected decision-making follows from administrative bloat. When the people making decisions about clinical workflows, scheduling ratios, documentation requirements, and care protocols are removed from clinical reality, those decisions tend to optimize for metrics that can be measured on a spreadsheet rather than for conditions that produce good clinical outcomes. A scheduling model that looks efficient from an administrative view can look impossible from a clinical view. The physician on the ground knows it doesn't work. But the feedback loop between clinical reality and administrative decision-making is often so attenuated that the knowledge never reaches the people with authority to change things.

Workforce depletion as an unacknowledged risk is the fourth finding, and it's the one with the most immediate consequence for the coming decade. The Permanente 2026 data on early exit trajectories isn't just a story about individual physicians. It's a population-level warning. When experienced, trained physicians exit clinical medicine ahead of schedule, what leaves with them is irreplaceable. Years of clinical judgment, subspecialty expertise, mentorship capacity, and institutional knowledge don't get backfilled with a new hire. They disappear. And they disappear at a moment when the U.S. physician shortage projections are already alarming.

The organizational diagnosis, then, is a system that is consuming its own workforce faster than it can replenish it, driven by incentive structures that prioritize short-term financial metrics over the long-term conditions that make medicine sustainable. It's not a mystery. It's a predictable outcome of a specific set of choices, made at the institutional and policy level, that have now been running long enough to produce measurable exit data.

Understanding this diagnosis matters for you personally, not just intellectually. When you understand that your exhaustion is a predictable response to a structurally dysfunctional system, a few things become possible that weren't possible before.

You stop spending energy blaming yourself. Burnout in a broken system isn't a character flaw. It's a signal. Your body and your mind are telling you that the conditions you're working in are past the threshold of what any person can sustain indefinitely. That signal deserves to be taken seriously rather than suppressed.

You start asking better questions. The question isn't "How do I get tougher?" or "How do I cope better?" The question is: "What, specifically, about my current situation is structural and therefore not fixable by my own effort alone? And what is actually within my control to change?" That question points you toward real options rather than toward another round of self-improvement in an unchanged environment.

You make better decisions about your future. Chapter 14 will walk you through the four-path triage model in detail, but the foundation of that model is an accurate assessment of your situation. You can't accurately assess your situation if you believe your distress is primarily a product of your own inadequacy. The Permanente 2026 data, the hassle factor research, and the organizational diagnosis in this chapter give you a factual basis for a different assessment: you are responding normally to an abnormal set of conditions.

That reframe doesn't tell you what to do next. That's what the rest of this book is for. But it clears the ground.

What This Means for Your Next Move

The system pathology chapter isn't here so you can feel validated and then return to the same situation. It's here because accurate diagnosis is the first requirement for effective action.

Before moving forward through this manual, do three things with what you've read here.

First, write down your own hassle factor inventory. Not your general feelings about your job. The specific, concrete sources of daily friction that consume your time and energy without producing clinical value. List them. Name them. Get them out of the ambient background noise and into a format you can actually analyze. Documentation burden. Approval processes. Meetings that could be emails. Inbox volume during off hours. Scheduling constraints you didn't set and can't control. Getting them on paper changes your relationship to them. They become external problems to be solved rather than internal failures to be endured.

Second, distinguish between structural and situational problems. Some of what's on your hassle factor list is structural: it's built into the institution, the specialty, the reimbursement model, or the regulatory environment. Changing it requires collective action, leverage, or exit. Some of it is situational: it's specific to your current employer, your current contract, your current department leadership. Situational problems can sometimes be addressed by negotiation, by changing roles, or by moving to a different practice environment. Knowing which is which matters enormously for deciding what action to take.

Third, look at the organizational diagnosis and honestly assess where your institution falls. Is decision-making connected to clinical reality, or is it made several layers above it? Are the incentives your employer is running on aligned with clinical quality, or primarily with margin and volume? Is the administrative structure there to support clinical work, or to administer it? Your answers don't determine your path, but they tell you how much structural resistance you're likely to meet if you try to improve your situation from within.

The chapters that follow build on this foundation. The inbox problem gets specific in Chapter 4. The tech paradox gets examined in Chapter 5. The corporate capture of medicine gets named in Chapter 6. And the practical framework for what you do about all of it starts in Chapter 11.

But the system pathology chapter is the one you come back to when leadership announces the next wellness initiative and you feel the familiar combination of exhaustion and rage. Come back to this chapter and remember: the research says you're right. The problem is structural. The solution has to be, too.

The Inbox That Ate Medicine

The inbox doesn't announce itself as a crisis. It just expands. Quietly, steadily, without anyone formally deciding it should become your second job. One day you're finishing your last patient note at 6 PM. The next you're triaging refill requests at 10 PM, then lab results at midnight, then prior auth appeals on Sunday morning. Nobody scheduled this. Nobody compensated you for it. It simply grew until it swallowed the edges of your life.

This is what the digital transformation of medicine actually delivered to practicing physicians: an always-open window into every clinical task that didn't fit inside the appointment slot. Patient portals were sold as a convenience. They became a pipeline. And that pipeline flows in one direction: toward you, around the clock, without additional pay, without clear limits, and without any institutional acknowledgment that it constitutes real work.

The message volume has exploded since the federal push for patient portal adoption. Practices that tracked inbox activity before and after portal implementation consistently report that physician message volume roughly doubled or more within a few years of going live. Patients aren't doing anything wrong by using the portals. They were told to. "Message your doctor." "Send your questions through the portal." "Check your results online." The system designed this behavior on purpose. Then it handed physicians the bill.

What nobody designed was a compensation model to match. The RVU system doesn't credit you for reading a patient's three-paragraph message about their knee pain, cross-referencing their medication list, crafting a response that avoids liability, and documenting the exchange. It doesn't credit you for the fifteen portal tasks stacked behind it. You do that work on your own time, unpaid, with the quiet understanding that if you don't, someone complains. Or something gets missed. Or the quality scores drop. So you do it.

That's the uncompensated labor problem in plain terms. The inbox became a second shift. The second shift has no overtime pay.

The Uncompensated Labor Problem

When healthcare systems talk about physician productivity, they almost always talk about patient volume. How many encounters did you complete? How many RVUs did you generate? The conversation almost never includes the hours spent after the last patient leaves.

Research on physician EHR use has consistently shown that for every hour spent in direct patient care, physicians spend a substantial portion of their day on EHR tasks outside of that clinical time. Some studies put the ratio at roughly one hour of EHR work for every two hours of patient contact. Others show primary care physicians spending more time on documentation and inbox management than on actual patient interaction across a full workday. The specific numbers shift depending on specialty and setting, but the pattern is universal: there is a documented, persistent, measurable gap between what the job description says and what the job actually requires.

The inbox sits at the center of that gap.

Portal messages, lab result reviews, prescription refills, specialist referral follow-ups, administrative task requests routed through clinical channels, nursing questions that got escalated because there wasn't a protocol, patient questions that arrived at 11 PM and are sitting in the queue when you log in at 6 AM. Every one of these items represents a clinical decision or a clinical communication. Every one carries a liability weight. And the institutional paycheck doesn't reflect any of them.

Some systems have started experimenting with charging patients a small fee for portal messages that require physician time, similar to a brief consultation charge. The results have been mixed. Patients sometimes reduce message volume. Billing infrastructure creates its own friction. Physicians rarely see that revenue anyway because it gets absorbed into overhead. The fundamental problem, which is that the work exists and someone has to do it, doesn't disappear. It just gets a different set of complications.

The honest framing is this: the inbox is labor. It requires clinical judgment. It carries malpractice risk. It takes time you don't get back. Calling it "asynchronous care" doesn't change what it is. It's a shift without a pay stub.

What makes it particularly grinding is the emotional texture of the work. A prior authorization appeal is frustrating but impersonal. An inbox message from a patient who is scared, angry, or in pain requires a different kind of attention. You're reading tone, making clinical judgments about urgency, managing the patient relationship, and drafting a response that's warm enough to hold the relationship, accurate enough to be medically sound, and brief enough that you might actually get through the next twelve items in the queue. That's skilled work. You'd never call it unskilled if a consultant were doing it and billing $400 an hour. But because it happens inside your EHR, it disappears into the institution's overhead.

Portal Aggression and the 24/7 Expectation

There's a particular category of inbox experience that physicians describe and that the research literature has started to capture. Patients who use the portal to express frustration, anger, or hostility in ways they'd never use face-to-face. It has a name now: portal aggression.

This isn't patients asking hard questions or advocating firmly for their care. Those exchanges can be difficult but they're clinically productive. Portal aggression is something different. It's the message that opens with a demand and closes with a threat. The message that questions your competence in three paragraphs. The message that copies your administrator and asks why you haven't responded in four hours on a Saturday. The message that arrives at 9 PM telling you your patient is done with you unless you respond tonight.

The screen creates a distance that lowers the threshold for hostility. Patients who would sit politely in an exam room and say "I've been worried about this" sometimes write something entirely different when they're alone with a phone and a text box.

There's no body language. There's no social accountability. There's just words, and whoever receives them has to manage their own response before deciding how to manage the clinical response.

That experience wears on you. Every physician who spends meaningful time in the inbox knows it. You learn to brace before you open certain threads. You start to feel something close to dread before your morning log-in. That dread is a real cost, and it doesn't appear anywhere in the wellness survey results your employer sends in a quarterly dashboard.

The 24/7 expectation compounds this. Portals don't have business hours. Patients send messages whenever it's convenient for them, which is rational from their perspective. The problem is that many institutions have established response-time expectations that de facto require physicians to check and answer messages outside of scheduled clinical time. A 24-hour response window sounds reasonable until you realize it means that a message sent at 5 PM on a Friday needs a physician response by 5 PM on Saturday. A message sent at 11 PM Thursday needs an answer before 11 PM Friday, which is likely a full clinic day.

Nobody put that in your job offer letter. Nobody told you during residency that patient portal management would become a significant portion of your weekly work. It arrived quietly, shaped by a combination of federal policy pushing for portal adoption, patient expectation calibrated by how quickly they can get responses in every other digital interaction in their lives, and institutional cultures that never drew a line about what physicians are actually responsible for.

The result is a job that has no real end time. You can leave the clinic. You can't leave the inbox.

Calculating Your Invisible Workload

Before you can negotiate anything, you need to know what you're actually dealing with. Most physicians have a rough sense that the inbox is a problem. Few have actually quantified how many hours per week it consumes. That number matters, because it's the foundation of any credible conversation with an employer about workload, compensation, or staffing.

Here's how to calculate your invisible workload with enough precision to be useful.

Start with a one-week log. For one representative week, track inbox activity separately from everything else. You're not logging clinic time, rounding time, or documentation time. Just the inbox: portal messages, lab result reviews, refill approvals, prescription prior auths routed through the EHR, referral coordination messages, and administrative tasks that arrived as clinical messages. Use a simple timer on your phone or a notebook. Round to the nearest five minutes. Don't try to be precise to the second. You're building a picture, not filing a timesheet.

Count the categories, not just the time. At the end of the week, sort your inbox activity into rough categories. Clinical decisions (anything requiring medical judgment), administrative tasks (forms, letters, prior auth paperwork), patient communications (portal messages requiring a drafted response), and system-generated noise (automated alerts, report flags, EHR notifications that don't require action but still require scanning). This breakdown matters because different categories have different solutions. Clinical decisions might need staffing support or protocol changes. Administrative tasks might be delegatable to trained non-physician staff. Patient communications might be reduceable through response templates or patient-facing FAQs.

Calculate the weekly total, then annualize it. If your one-week log shows eight hours of inbox work outside of scheduled clinical time, that's approximately 400 hours per year. At a conservative physician hourly rate, you can put a dollar value on that time. That number is what you bring to a negotiation. It's not a complaint. It's a calculation.

Compare it to what's documented in your job description. Many physician employment agreements don't mention inbox management at all. They describe clinical hours, call schedules, and administrative duties in general terms. If your job description doesn't include the inbox, you have a documented gap between what you were hired for and what the job actually requires. That gap is a negotiating lever.

Note what you're skipping. In a week of logging, you'll likely also notice the tasks you're deprioritizing or delaying because the inbox volume is too high. That's important data too. Unreviewed results. Delayed responses. Work you're pushing to tomorrow because today was already full. This isn't a record of your failures. It's a record of system overload.

The point of this exercise isn't to make you feel worse about how much you're doing. You probably already know it's a lot. The point is to convert a felt experience into a documented fact. Feelings get dismissed. Numbers get a response.

What Is Actually Negotiable

Here's what most physicians don't know because nobody told them: the inbox is negotiable. Not perfectly, not immediately, and not without friction. But pieces of it can be shifted, delegated, restructured, or reduced. The assumption that you're personally responsible for every digital task that arrives in your EHR is an institutional preference, not a legal or clinical mandate.

Let's go through the categories of inbox work and what's actually on the table.

Prescription refills. In most states and most practice settings, trained medical assistants or licensed nurses can process routine refills on stable, established medications under a physician-reviewed protocol. You set the parameters. They execute. You review and sign. That process is already in place in many practices. If it's not in yours, it's a reasonable request to make. The alternative is that you personally approve every maintenance refill for every chronic patient, which can consume a surprising portion of your daily inbox volume. Pull up your refill queue and count how many items are for patients on medications they've been on for years with no complications. Those shouldn't require your full clinical attention every time.

Lab result routing. Normal results on stable patients don't require a physician-drafted message. Many EHR systems can auto-release normal results with a templated message explaining what "normal" means in plain language. Abnormal results still need your eyes. But the volume of normal result notifications that currently land in your inbox and require some form of acknowledgment or routing can often be handled through protocol. Ask your informatics team what the options are. If they say the system doesn't support it, ask what system it would take to support it. Put it in writing.

After-hours portal messages. Your institution may have established a response-time expectation without ever getting your formal agreement to it. Check your employment contract and your employee handbook. If there's no written standard, there's room to propose one. A reasonable standard for non-urgent portal messages is a response within two business days, consistent with how most other professional communications are handled. That doesn't mean patients in distress wait two days. It means the message asking whether it's okay to take ibuprofen with their blood pressure medication doesn't need a midnight response.

Message triage by clinical staff. In a well-structured practice, your medical assistant or nurse reviews incoming portal messages before they ever reach you. They flag genuinely urgent items, route administrative items to the appropriate staff, answer questions that fall within their scope using approved templates, and batch-deliver the clinically relevant items to you in a structured way rather than as a constant drip. This isn't a new idea. Many specialties have used message triage protocols for years. If your practice hasn't implemented one, that's a staffing and workflow gap, not an inevitability.

The 24/7 expectation itself. If your institution has published a patient-facing policy that promises same-day portal responses, that policy was created by administrators and marketing, not by physicians. It can be revised. It should be revised, because it sets patient expectations that create the hostile tone when responses don't arrive in two hours. A realistic, transparent patient-facing communication policy, something like "your care team responds to portal messages within two business days," protects both patients and physicians. Patients know what to expect. You're not managing the fallout from unmet promises you never made.

Your own response habits. Some of the inbox volume is genuinely structural and needs institutional solutions. Some of it is a pattern you've developed. Checking the inbox at 10 PM because you didn't want it waiting for you in the morning. Responding to every message the same day because you're not sure which ones can wait. Drafting long, detailed responses to questions that could be answered in two sentences because you're managing anticipated follow-up questions. None of these habits are character flaws. They developed for understandable reasons. They can also be changed, deliberately, with some structure.

Response templates are underused by most physicians. For the questions that come up repeatedly, a well-crafted two-paragraph response that you can copy, personalize in one sentence, and send handles the clinical need without requiring you to write from scratch every time. You're not being impersonal. You're being efficient about the parts of the work that don't require fresh thinking.

Batching also helps. Checking and responding to inbox messages twice a day, at specific times, is more cognitively sustainable than responding reactively throughout the day. The constant context-switching between patient care and inbox management is one of the reasons the inbox feels more exhausting than the total time would suggest. Every switch costs attention. Batching reduces switches.

Your Next Move

Start with the one-week log this week. Not after your next vacation or after the end of the quarter. This week. You need real numbers from your real inbox, not a general impression.

When the week is done, sort your total inbox hours into the categories above. Then identify the single highest-volume item that could reasonably be delegated or protocolized with proper staff support. Pick one. Bring a concrete proposal to your practice manager, not a complaint about being overwhelmed, but a specific workflow change with a clear description of who would do what differently.

If you're employed by a large health system, check whether your contract or employee handbook specifies inbox response-time expectations. If it does, you have something specific to negotiate around. If it doesn't, you have grounds to establish a written standard rather than operating on an implicit expectation that's never been defined and therefore can never be pushed back on.

One more thing worth sitting with. The fact that you've been absorbing this workload without complaint probably looks like loyalty or professionalism from the outside. From your side of the screen, it's exhaustion. The institution didn't create the inbox problem out of malice. It created it out of inertia, because nobody made it expensive enough to fix. Making it visible, documenting it, and bringing it to the table as a business problem rather than a personal struggle is how that inertia gets interrupted.

You don't owe the system unlimited digital availability. You owe your patients good clinical care. Those two things stopped being the same when the inbox became a second shift. Naming that difference is where the work begins.

The Tech Paradox

The pitch sounded like a rescue mission.

Artificial intelligence, the vendors promised, would give medicine back to physicians. Smart ambient scribes would eliminate the documentation grind. Predictive algorithms would flag the sick patients before they crashed. Automated prior auth tools would cut through the insurance wall. The inbox problem, the charting problem, the "you spend more time looking at a screen than at a patient" problem — all of it, solvable. Just buy the platform.

Some of it even worked.

Documentation burnout among physicians who adopted ambient AI scribe tools dropped from 51.9% to 38.8%. That's a real number and a real reduction. If you've spent years dictating into an EHR at 10 p.m., watching a tool absorb a patient visit and generate a coherent note in real time feels close to miraculous. The administrative weight on that task lightens. The cursor stops blinking at you accusingly.

But pajama time is still at 20.9%.

Physicians are still doing nearly a fifth of their clinical work after hours, in their homes, on personal devices, after the official workday has ended. The scribe caught the note. The inbox still didn't empty. The prior auth still needed a human to fight it. The patient portal still lit up at 9 p.m. with a question that felt urgent to the sender and medically mundane to you but still required a response because the metric that tracks response time doesn't care what else you had going on that evening.

That's the tech paradox in plain language. The tools that actually work tend to solve the easiest part of the problem. The harder part (who has authority over your schedule, your workload, your clinical decisions, and your time) those tools don't touch. And the vendors don't advertise that limitation.

The AI Scribe Dividend

Let's be clear about what ambient AI scribes actually do well, because dismissing them entirely would be dishonest and would leave money on the table.

Documentation is one of the most time-intensive and least clinically meaningful tasks a physician performs in a typical day. You know the medicine. You made the diagnosis. You formed the plan. Then you spent twenty minutes converting that thinking into structured documentation language that satisfies billing requirements, liability standards, and accreditation checklists. The clinical value of that documentation to the patient is close to zero. Its administrative and legal value is enormous. That mismatch has been grinding physicians down for years.

An ambient scribe changes the equation. You speak naturally with a patient during the visit. The system listens, processes the conversation, and produces a structured clinical note. You review, edit, approve. Time spent: a fraction of what it took before. The cognitive load of switching between the patient in front of you and the documentation requirements hanging over the visit drops significantly.

The 13-point reduction in documentation burnout (from 51.9% to 38.8%) reflects that relief. It's not a rounding error. For physicians who were approaching the edge, that reduction in friction can extend a career, improve visit quality, and genuinely restore some of the presence that documentation demands had stolen.

So yes: if your institution offers an ambient scribe tool and you haven't tried it, try it. If you're negotiating a new contract and tech access is on the table, ask specifically about ambient documentation support. If you're running your own practice, cost out the tools and compare them against what your charting time is actually worth at your hourly rate.

The dividend is real. The error is assuming the dividend solves the underlying problem.

Why Technology Does Not Fix Autonomy Deficits

Here's what the tech sales cycle never mentions. The burnout driving most physician exits isn't primarily about documentation load. Documentation is a symptom. The disease is loss of control.

Physicians cite three core drivers of burnout more consistently than any others. They report too many bureaucratic tasks. They report a loss of autonomy over clinical decisions. And they report that the work has stopped feeling meaningful because the system has reorganized their role from clinician to data-entry node. Documentation is a bureaucratic task, yes. But the other two drivers — autonomy loss and meaning erosion — don't respond to AI scribes. They don't respond to any software.

When a hospitalist can't discharge a patient without administrator approval tied to a length-of-stay metric, no technology fixes that. When a primary care physician faces a prior authorization process that requires a peer-to-peer call to justify a medication they've prescribed safely for years, no EHR upgrade changes that equation. When a specialist sees productivity pressure expressed as a daily RVU target that leaves no margin for complex patients who need more time, a faster documentation tool just means you can see more patients in the same window — which compounds the problem rather than solving it.

Technology optimized for throughput in a broken system produces more throughput in a broken system. That's not progress. It's acceleration toward the same wall.

The physicians who feel the most deceived by the tech promise aren't the ones who hated the tools. Many of them liked the tools. They're the ones who implemented the tools faithfully, saw the documentation metrics improve, and then realized nothing else had changed. The inbox was still there. The staffing shortages were still there. The administrator with the spreadsheet was still there. The ambient scribe made their evenings 30 minutes shorter and their days 20 patients longer.

That's the bait-and-switch. Sell efficiency. Pocket the gains. Leave the physician no better off in terms of the thing that actually matters: do they have meaningful control over how they practice medicine?

Pajama Time at 20.9%

The 20.9% figure deserves more attention than it gets, because it's a quiet indictment of every technology investment healthcare organizations have made in the last decade.

Nearly one in five hours of physician work happens after hours, outside the clinic, on personal time. This is work without boundaries. It's the refill requests that stack up between patient visits and get addressed at night. It's the lab results that come back at 7 p.m. and need review before they become a gap in care. It's the portal messages from patients who couldn't reach anyone during business hours and sent their questions into the queue. It's the documentation that didn't get finished because the afternoon ran long and there was no buffer built into the schedule.

Pajama time has persisted through multiple waves of EHR upgrades, multiple generations of clinical decision support tools, multiple rounds of inbox management training, and now the first wave of ambient AI scribes. It doesn't move much. That consistency is telling.

The reason it won't go away with technology alone is structural. After-hours work exists because the official hours have been overpacked. Physicians are scheduled at a density that doesn't allow for complete task resolution during the workday. The asynchronous communication tools that were supposed to reduce burden — the patient portal chief among them — instead created a new channel of demand that operates on patient timelines, not physician schedules. And patients didn't reduce their expectations when the portal launched. They expanded them.

So the math works like this: overpacked daytime schedule creates spillover. Spillover fills the evening. Evening work tools are convenient, so evening work expands to fill available time. The technology that was supposed to eliminate pajama time is now the mechanism through which pajama time happens. The phone that lets you review a chart from your couch is also the phone that makes it impossible to stop reviewing charts from your couch.

Organizations know this. They track after-hours EHR access in their burnout dashboards. Some of them put it in presentations. Very few of them change the scheduling density that causes it, because scheduling density is tied directly to productivity targets and revenue projections. The pajama time data is descriptive. The causes are financial.

And that's where the tech conversation hits its ceiling. You can give a physician a better tool for doing the work. You can't use a tool to fix an organization's decision to require more work than working hours can hold.

Informed Optimism: Using Tech Without Being Deceived by It

None of this means you should refuse to use the available tools or assume they're worthless because they don't solve everything. Informed optimism is the useful position here. Take the real gains. Know their limits. Don't let anyone sell you a tool as a solution to a problem the tool can't touch.

There are specific things technology can help you with right now, and being tactical about each one matters.

Ambient documentation tools are the clearest win. If you're spending more than 90 minutes per day on charting and documentation review, a well-implemented ambient scribe will likely return 30 to 60 minutes of that time. That's time you can redirect to patients, to rest, or to the boundary work later chapters cover in detail. The tool earns its place if it genuinely reduces after-hours chart completion. If it just makes it easier to see more patients in the same day because administration notices the documentation speed, you've been handed a productivity trap disguised as a relief measure. Track your own before-and-after data. Look specifically at whether your pajama time drops, not just your per-note time.

Inbox management tools vary widely. The best of them help you triage message priority, auto-route administrative questions to the right team member, and create standing reply templates for common queries. The worst of them add a layer of complexity without reducing volume. Before adopting any inbox tool, ask the vendor one question: what happens to total message volume after implementation? If they can't answer with data, they're selling a workflow gadget, not a volume solution.

Predictive analytics and clinical decision support tools are genuinely useful when they surface relevant information in the moment of care and stay out of the way the rest of the time. When they generate alerts you can't act on, for patients whose risk factors you already know, at a rate that turns every screen into a noise machine, they don't reduce your cognitive load. They add to it. Alert fatigue is a documented problem that worsens physician performance and increases error rates. Every organization has overconfigured their alert systems at some point. You have the right to bring data on alert burden to your department leadership and ask for a formal review of which alerts are firing most often and which are generating the most overrides. Alerts that physicians override 80% of the time are noise. Noise is not neutral. It costs attention.

Scheduling tools and patient flow optimization deserve a separate look because they sit at the intersection of technology and the autonomy deficit. When scheduling algorithms are controlled by administrators optimizing for slot utilization, those tools work against you. When you have input into scheduling structure — visit length, buffer slots, message response windows built into the day — those same categories of tools can be configured to protect you. The technology isn't the variable. The variable is who controls the configuration.

This is the question worth asking about every tech platform your institution rolls out: who controls the settings? If the answer is an operations team optimizing for throughput, the tool will likely extract more from you regardless of what the marketing materials say about physician wellness. If the settings are negotiable, you have leverage worth using.

What Smart Adoption Actually Looks Like

Physicians who get real benefit from technology tend to share a few habits worth adopting.

They evaluate tools based on after-hours time, not on-shift speed. A tool that makes you faster during clinic hours matters less than a tool that gets you off the EHR by 7 p.m. Set your own baseline before implementing anything. Track your pajama time for two weeks. Then implement. Then track again. The data you generate about your own workflow is the only data that matters for your decision.

They negotiate access before adoption. If your contract or employment arrangement is being updated and your organization is pushing a new platform, ask whether ambient scribe access, inbox management support, or after-hours EHR load reduction targets are written into your agreement. Many physicians don't think to negotiate tech support as a contract term. It's as legitimate as call frequency or CME allowance.

They separate the tool from the policy. This is critical. An ambient scribe is a tool. The policy that determines how many patients you see per day is a management decision. These two things are not connected, but administrators often present them together — as in "we're giving you this efficiency tool so we can optimize your panel size." The tool is yours to use or not use on its own merits. The panel size decision is a separate negotiation. Don't let the delivery of a tool function as implicit consent to an increased workload.

They build manual overrides into their workflow. Technology fails. Systems go down. The AI-generated note needs editing. Treating any platform as infallible creates a new vulnerability. Keeping your own documentation habits functional, even when the scribe is doing the heavy lifting, protects you when the tool breaks and protects you from over-delegating clinical accuracy to an automated system that doesn't carry malpractice exposure.

They report alert fatigue formally. When a clinical decision support tool is generating alerts that are mostly noise, that's a patient safety issue, a physician wellness issue, and an organizational efficiency problem all at once. You don't have to tolerate it quietly. Logging alert overrides, tracking response patterns, and bringing the data to a department meeting or patient safety committee turns a private frustration into a fixable institutional problem.

The Honest Summary

Technology is a legitimate part of the answer to physician burnout. The documentation relief from ambient AI scribes is measurable and real. Clinical decision support, when configured well, improves patient care and reduces cognitive burden. Tools that help manage inbox volume can claw back time that would otherwise disappear into evenings and weekends.

But pajama time is still 20.9%. And it will stay close to that number as long as organizations continue to treat efficiency gains as justification for higher throughput. Every time technology makes a physician faster, an organization faces a choice: let the physician have that time back, or add more work to fill the gap. The consistent pattern across healthcare settings has been to add more work.

That's not a technology problem. It's a values and power problem. Who decides how the efficiency dividend gets distributed? Right now, in most healthcare organizations, it's not the physician.

The tools are worth using strategically. Approach them the way you'd approach any clinical intervention. Ask what the evidence shows. Ask what the mechanism of action is. Ask what the side effects are and who controls them. Know the difference between a symptom relief and a cure.

Documentation burnout dropped 13 points with ambient scribes. That's symptom relief. The autonomy deficit that causes burnout to persist regardless of documentation speed is structural. Fixing it requires the approaches in Part III of this book: negotiating boundaries, building financial leverage, and making a clear-eyed decision about whether your current environment can be repaired or whether it needs to be left.

Technology can help you survive the day. Structural change is what determines whether the day is worth surviving.

Your next move: For one week, track your after-hours EHR time in 15-minute increments. Note what tasks fill that time: charting, inbox, refills, lab review, or other. At the end of the week, you'll have a clear picture of where pajama time actually comes from in your practice. That breakdown tells you which tools are worth evaluating and which structural changes are non-negotiable. A tool that eliminates charting at 10 p.m. helps if charting is 80% of your after-hours load. It doesn't help if inbox and refills are the real drivers. Know your data before the next vendor walks through your door.

From Profession to Production Line

Something shifted in American medicine around the time hospital systems started calling their doctors "providers." The word arrived quietly in policy documents, then insurance forms, then the hallway conversations of administrators who'd never held a stethoscope. Most physicians noticed it and said nothing. A few pushed back and were told they were being sensitive. The rest filed it away alongside all the other small indignities that stack up in a career.

That word change wasn't accidental. It was a business decision.

This chapter is about how medicine got turned into a production line, who built it, what it cost physicians, and how to spot the machinery operating inside your own institution. Because you can't protect yourself from something you haven't named. And most physicians are so deep inside the system they've stopped seeing the walls.

The Private Equity Playbook

Private equity didn't stumble into healthcare. It targeted it.

The logic is straightforward from a financial standpoint. Healthcare is a sector with reliable demand, fragmented ownership, and historically poor business management. Independent physician practices, built by clinicians who went to medical school instead of business school, had real revenue and almost no sophistication around deal structures. That combination looked like opportunity to investors whose job is to find undervalued assets and extract returns.

The playbook works in stages. First, a PE firm acquires a founding or anchor practice, usually offering the physician-owners a significant cash payout. That payout is attractive. Many physicians carry student loan debt, delayed earnings from long training years, and a reasonable desire to reduce financial risk. The offer looks like relief.

After the anchor acquisition, the firm moves fast. It buys adjacent practices in the same specialty and geography, building what the industry calls a "platform." The platform creates market scale. Scale creates pricing leverage with insurers. Pricing leverage creates margin. And margin is what gets sold when the firm exits, usually within five to seven years.

That exit window matters more than almost anything else in this story. PE firms don't hold assets indefinitely. They're structured to sell. Which means every decision made during ownership is filtered through the question of what maximizes the sale price. That's not clinical logic. It's financial logic. And those two things are frequently at war with each other.

The cost optimization part of the model is where physicians feel the squeeze. After acquisition, the pressure to increase volume is immediate. More patients, shorter visits, tighter scheduling templates. Overhead gets cut. Support staff gets reduced or replaced with lower-cost alternatives. In many specialties, the ratio of advanced practice providers to physicians shifts sharply. Not because the clinical model demands it, but because the financial model does.

Physicians inside these structures often describe a specific moment when they realized the deal had changed them. It's not dramatic. It's the scheduling template that adds two patients per hour with no explanation. It's the productivity metric that appears in a dashboard they didn't ask for. It's the meeting where someone from corporate talks about "throughput" and nobody in the room flinches except them.

The specialties hit hardest by private equity acquisition include emergency medicine, anesthesiology, dermatology, gastroenterology, ophthalmology, and urology. These are high-volume, procedurally oriented fields with predictable revenue streams.

But primary care has increasingly entered the target zone as insurers and health systems work to control referral networks from the front door.

The physicians who sold often had no idea what they were signing. Chapter 9 goes into the contract mechanics in detail. The short version: the fine print in most PE acquisition agreements includes provisions that shift clinical and administrative control to management entities in ways that aren't obvious at signing. Physicians retain their license. They give up almost everything else.

Vertical Integration and What It Costs Physicians

Private equity is one arm of corporate capture. Vertical integration by large health systems is the other.

Vertical integration means a single organization owns multiple levels of the care delivery chain. A large hospital system buys primary care practices to control patient referrals into its network. It then acquires specialty groups to keep those referrals in-house. It adds urgent care, imaging, pharmacy, and post-acute care. The goal is to keep every dollar a patient spends within the system's walls.

From a market standpoint, this creates something close to a local monopoly in many regions. When a health system employs the majority of physicians in a geographic area, physicians have fewer places to work, less leverage to negotiate, and fewer options when conditions become intolerable.

This is the part that rarely gets said clearly in wellness workshops: the reason physicians feel trapped isn't a mindset problem. It's a market structure problem. When consolidation has narrowed your real employment alternatives to one or two large systems, the power balance between you and your employer shifts dramatically. They can set the terms. And they do.

The employed physician model, which now covers the majority of practicing clinicians in the United States, came with promises. Stability. Benefits. Freedom from the administrative burden of running an independent practice. Many of those promises were genuine at first. The problem is that employment transforms the clinical relationship into an employment relationship. And employment relationships are governed by the interests of the employer, not the professional standards of the employee.

What vertical integration costs physicians specifically:

It costs clinical autonomy. When you're employed by a system whose revenue depends on keeping patients within its network, referrals outside that network become problematic. You may not be told not to refer out. You'll simply be tracked on whether you do. The pressure is there in the data, in the dashboard, in the quarterly review conversation that mentions your "network utilization."

It costs schedule control. Employed physicians in large systems typically have limited authority over their own scheduling templates. The template is set by administrators who are optimizing for room utilization and provider productivity, two metrics that have nothing to do with clinical quality or physician sustainability.

It costs exit options. Noncompete clauses are common in employed physician contracts. These clauses restrict where a physician can practice within a defined geography for a defined period after leaving. In a consolidated market, those restrictions can effectively mean starting over somewhere new or waiting out the clock. The practical effect is that leaving becomes a much higher-stakes decision than it should be. That leverage is not accidental.

The standard defense of vertical integration is that it creates efficiency and improves care coordination. In some cases, coordination does improve. But efficiency in a corporate healthcare context usually means lower cost per unit of service. And the unit of service is you seeing a patient. If seeing that patient takes 15 minutes instead of 20 because the template demands it, the system has achieved its efficiency goal whether or not you had enough time to actually do the job well.

The Language of Devaluation

Language isn't decoration. It's a tool. And in corporate healthcare, the language shift from "physician" to "provider" was a tool used with precision.

"Provider" is an insurance billing category. It encompasses physicians, nurse practitioners, physician assistants, certified registered nurse anesthetists, and others who deliver clinical services. From a payer standpoint, collapsing all of these into a single label simplifies contracts and reimbursement structures. From a management standpoint, it also does something else: it erases the distinction between twelve years of post-graduate training and two.

That erasure has financial consequences for physicians. When a hospital system can market its "providers" without distinguishing between credential levels, it creates price competition within its own workforce. It can hire a nurse practitioner at a fraction of a physician's salary and bill at 85% of the physician rate. The math on that is obvious. The clinical implications are a conversation health systems prefer not to have publicly.

The physician-to-provider shift also does something more subtle. It strips the word "physician" of its professional weight. A profession implies a set of standards, obligations, and autonomy that exist independent of any employer. A provider implies a functional role within a service delivery system. Professions have ethics boards, licensure standards, and legal frameworks that protect both the professional and the public. Providers have job descriptions.

When your employer calls you a provider, they're not just using shorthand. They're signaling something about how they see the relationship. You are a unit in their delivery model. Your professional identity is adjacent to, but separate from, your economic function in their organization. That framing gives them more flexibility to manage you the way they'd manage any other labor cost.

Watch for the downstream effects of this language in your own workplace. If the scheduling system refers to you as a "provider slot," if your performance reviews measure "provider productivity," if your department is called a "clinical services unit" rather than a medical department, those are signals. The language reflects the underlying business logic.

The word "physician" matters. Use it about yourself. Require others to use it about you when the clinical credential is relevant. This isn't ego. It's accuracy. And it's a small act of professional self-defense in an environment that benefits from blurring the distinction.

The language problem extends beyond the provider/physician binary. Corporate healthcare has developed a vocabulary designed to make clinical work sound like manufacturing. Patients become "encounters." Appointments become "units of service." Clinical judgment becomes "variance from protocol." Efficiency becomes the primary metric, and everything that can't be easily measured gets deprioritized.

When medicine becomes a manufacturing process in language, it becomes easier to manage it like one. Physicians are then workers on a line, expected to hit throughput targets, reduce variance, and minimize cost per unit. The fact that the units are human beings with complicated lives doesn't fit neatly into that framework. So it gets left out.

Recognizing Corporate Capture in Your Own Institution

Most physicians inside a captured institution don't experience a dramatic moment of recognition. The capture happens gradually, through accumulated small changes that each seem individually manageable. The template gets tighter. The metric dashboard expands. A committee that used to be physician-led gets a new administrator co-chair. A policy change arrives via email rather than through shared governance. None of these feel like a hostile takeover. Taken together, they describe one.

Here's a working list of signs that corporate capture is operating in your institution. These are patterns, not diagnostic criteria. You're likely to recognize several of them.

Governance erosion. Physician leadership positions become advisory rather than decision-making. The medical executive committee makes recommendations; administration makes decisions. Committee chairs are appointed rather than elected. Physicians are invited to "provide input" on decisions that have already been made.

Metric proliferation. New dashboards appear tracking your productivity, your door-to-discharge time, your patient satisfaction scores, your referral patterns, your after-visit call-back rates. Some of these metrics are clinically meaningful. Many aren't. The common feature is that they're tracked, reported to your supervisor, and woven into compensation or performance reviews. The message is clear: you are being watched against targets you didn't set.

APP substitution without clinical rationale. Your department adds advanced practice providers at a faster rate than it adds physicians. The stated reason is usually workforce availability or cost. The actual driver is often the margin differential. If this is happening in your department, look at whether APP-to-physician supervision ratios have expanded beyond what you're clinically comfortable with. That ratio has liability implications that eventually land on you, not the administrator who set the staffing model.

Communication hierarchies that exclude physicians. Administrative decisions affecting clinical operations get made in meetings physicians don't attend. You learn about policy changes through email after implementation. When you raise concerns, you're directed to a formal feedback channel that documents your concern without changing the outcome.

Noncompete clauses and tail coverage shifts. Employment contracts include restrictions that limit your exit options. Tail coverage for malpractice is shifted to the departing physician. Signing bonuses include clawback provisions that make leaving in the first two or three years financially painful. The financial structure of your employment is designed to raise the cost of leaving.

Quality metrics weaponized as productivity proxies. Your HEDIS scores or quality metrics are framed as performance evaluations rather than improvement tools. If you score below a threshold, your compensation takes a hit. The metrics themselves may be legitimate. Using them as a stick to pressure higher volume is not.

The consultant visit. A firm hired to analyze "operational efficiency" interviews clinical staff and then recommends changes to scheduling templates, staffing ratios, or service lines. Physicians are consulted during the process and ignored in the output. The recommendations consistently favor higher volume and lower labor cost.

None of these signs in isolation means your institution is beyond repair. Some are present in almost every large health system. The question is whether they're being addressed through genuine shared governance or whether physician input is theater while decisions are made elsewhere.

The way to find out is to test it. Raise a specific clinical concern through official channels. Document the response. Note whether the concern is engaged substantively or redirected. Notice whether raising it has any social or professional cost. The answer to those questions tells you more about your institution than any mission statement does.

What You Can Actually Do Right Now

Understanding corporate capture is useful. Being able to act on that understanding is what this book is for.

The first practical step is a clear-eyed audit of your current situation. Not a crisis inventory, just an honest look at four things.

Who actually controls your schedule? If you can adjust your own template, you have leverage. If your template is set by someone who doesn't see patients, you don't. Know which one is true for you, because it determines what tools are available in your next negotiation.

What does your contract actually say about noncompetes and tail coverage? If you haven't read your employment agreement recently, read it this week. Pull the specific noncompete radius and duration. Find the tail coverage provision. Find the termination-without-cause clause and its notice period. These numbers will matter if you decide to leave, and knowing them now means you won't be surprised later.

Who holds physician leadership positions in your institution, and how were they selected? If your department chief or CMO was appointed by administration rather than elected by the medical staff, that tells you something about how governance actually functions. It doesn't mean those individuals are bad actors. It means the structure gives them limited ability to protect physician interests when those interests conflict with organizational priorities.

What would it take for you to leave? This is the question most physicians haven't answered because it feels disloyal or defeatist. It's neither. Knowing your actual exit conditions is how you maintain leverage inside a system. Chapter 9 covers the financial side of this in detail and Chapter 13 walks through building your runway. The point here is simply: if you've never asked yourself what it would take, you don't know whether you're staying by choice or by default.

Corporate capture works best on physicians who believe they have no options. Every tool in Part III of this book is designed to change that belief by giving you real, operational options rather than theoretical ones.

The production line model depends on your compliance. It depends on you staying quiet when the template tightens. It depends on you absorbing the extra inbox messages and the extra documentation without complaint. It depends on you not knowing what your contract says, not knowing your financial runway, and not knowing your rights within medical staff bylaws.

Naming the model doesn't fix it. But physicians who can see the machinery clearly make different decisions than physicians who believe their exhaustion is a personal failure. The machinery is real. The exhaustion is a rational response to working inside it.

That's where this chapter lands: what you're experiencing isn't a performance problem. It's a structural problem that benefits from your silence. The next chapters in this section cover how the academic world runs its own version of the same capture, how gender compounds the damage, and how the contract itself was written to protect the institution rather than you.

You're not imagining the production line. You're working on it.

The Ivory Tower Trap and Toxic Calling Culture

The offer sounds generous. A faculty appointment, a research allocation, the chance to teach the next generation, and the prestige of a university affiliation. Academic medicine sells a compelling package, and for many physicians leaving residency, it's the destination. The promise is simple: trade some income for meaning, intellectual community, and freedom to shape your own work.

What the offer doesn't include is the fine print.

Academic Medicine's Hidden Contract

Academic medicine runs on a concept called the "three-legged stool." Clinical work. Research. Teaching. The idea is that all three legs support each other, that the combination creates a richer professional life than any single track alone.

The reality is that you're doing three jobs. Usually for the salary of one.

New faculty learn this quickly. Clinical loads aren't lighter just because you have a faculty title. In most academic medical centers, the RVU demands on junior attendings rival community practice, sometimes exceed it. The difference is that you're also expected to write grants, mentor students, publish, sit on committees, and contribute to departmental education. All of that happens in the same 24-hour day.

The research allocation is often the cruelest part. A new faculty member might receive 20% protected time for scholarship. In practice, that protection evaporates the moment the department needs clinical coverage. A colleague calls in sick. A scheduling gap appears. The chair sends an email asking if you can "just cover" one more session this week. You do it, because you're a team player, because you want tenure, because you don't want to be seen as difficult.

That 20% becomes 10%. Then zero. The grant deadlines don't move.

Teaching carries its own weight. Running small groups, supervising residents in clinic, providing feedback on student write-ups — all of it is expected, most of it is underpaid relative to actual time invested. "Teaching is part of the mission" is the phrase used to justify the gap between what you do and what you're compensated for doing.

The hidden contract in academic medicine isn't written anywhere. It's transmitted through culture. You learn it by watching senior faculty absorb impossible workloads without complaint. You learn it in the way people look at you if you ask about protected time enforcement or salary equity. You learn it when you realize that "joining the mission" is institutional shorthand for accepting whatever conditions exist without negotiating them.

This isn't unique to one institution. It's structural. Academic medicine depends on a steady supply of physicians who believe the prestige and meaning of the work justify the terms. The system doesn't need to be explicit about its exploitation because the culture polices itself.

The junior physician who arrived full of excitement about research and teaching gradually becomes someone managing three incompatible jobs with a smile, hoping the next promotion cycle rewards their patience. Sometimes it does. Often it doesn't. And in the meantime, the system gets years of output that wouldn't have been possible if the actual terms had been stated clearly at the start.

That's the hidden contract. It works because the people inside it often don't see it until they're already deep in.

KOLs Weaponizing the Privilege of Medicine

Key Opinion Leaders, or KOLs, are a fixture of academic medicine. They're the department chairs, the named professors, the conference keynote speakers, the physicians whose names appear on major clinical guidelines. They carry real authority in the profession. Their opinions shape training, policy, and culture.

They're also, in many cases, the primary enforcers of the status quo.

KOLs didn't invent the "privilege of medicine" argument, but many deploy it with precision. The argument goes like this: medicine is a privilege, not a right. You were chosen from thousands of applicants. You have skills no one else has. Patients trust you with their lives. To complain about your working conditions is to betray that trust, to elevate your comfort over your patients' needs, to reveal that you never really understood what medicine was about.

It's a powerful argument. It works because it contains a grain of truth. Medicine does involve real privilege. The training, the relationships, the ability to help people at the worst moments of their lives — that's genuinely meaningful. Nobody who went into medicine for the right reasons would deny it.

But weaponizing that truth to suppress legitimate grievances is a manipulation. Full stop.

When a KOL lectures residents about "entitlement" for asking about work-hour limits, that's not wisdom. When a department chair dismisses concerns about unsustainable patient volumes by reminding staff that "this is what we signed up for," that's not leadership. When a senior physician tells a colleague considering leaving that they're "abandoning their patients" or "wasting their training," that's not mentorship. It's pressure. It's a way of using the genuine meaning of medicine as a lever to extract compliance.

The KOL version of this argument is especially effective because it comes from inside the profession. When a hospital administrator tells you to be grateful, you can recognize that as corporate messaging. When a physician you deeply respect says the same thing, it's harder to dismiss. It has the weight of experience, of authority, of someone who presumably knows what medicine is really about.

That's exactly why it lands so hard. And why it needs to be named clearly.

The physicians making these arguments often built their careers in a different era. Research funding was more available. Tenure meant something. Clinical loads were genuinely more manageable. Autonomy was the norm. The ivory tower, for them, was actually insulated from the market pressures that define medicine today.

They're not entirely wrong about what medicine used to be. They're giving advice suited to a world that no longer exists. And when they use that advice to tell you that your exhaustion is a character flaw rather than a reasonable response to an unsustainable system, they're doing harm.

The insulation is the core problem. KOLs at major academic centers often have endowed chairs, named professorships, administrative support, negotiated clinical loads, and grant infrastructure that bear no resemblance to front-line practice. They may not have personally dealt with an insurance prior authorization in years. Their inbox looks nothing like yours. When they speak about the rewards of medicine, they're often describing a version of the job that you've never had access to.

Their experience is real. It just isn't yours. And it definitely isn't evidence that your experience is wrong.

There's also an incentive problem worth naming. KOLs who've risen through academic hierarchies have strong personal reasons to defend those hierarchies. If the system is functioning well enough to elevate people like them, the system can't be as broken as the front-line physicians are saying. Acknowledging systemic dysfunction means acknowledging that their own rise might have involved conditions that were unfair to others. That's uncomfortable. It's easier to attribute other people's struggles to attitude.

None of this means every senior physician who invokes medicine's meaning is acting in bad faith. Many genuinely believe what they're saying. But belief doesn't soften the impact. A culture that uses medicine's nobility to silence legitimate complaints does damage regardless of whether the people doing it are sincere.

The Vocation Trap

The word "vocation" comes from the Latin for "calling." Medicine has always carried that framing. You're not just doing a job, you're answering a call. The call came with years of sacrifice, with debt, with delayed relationships and postponed financial stability, and with the understanding that all of it was worth it because medicine isn't just a career. It's a purpose.

That framing is emotionally true for a lot of physicians. Most people who go into medicine feel genuine pull toward the work. Helping people, solving complex problems, being trusted with something sacred — these aren't manufactured feelings. They're real.

The problem is what happens when institutions discover that the "calling" framing is financially convenient.

A physician who sees medicine as a calling will tolerate conditions that a physician who sees it as a job would never accept. That's not a character flaw. It's a predictable consequence of how meaning gets tied to endurance. If this is your calling, then suffering through it becomes a sign of commitment rather than a signal that something is broken. Complaining starts to feel like complaining about your own values.

Institutions learned this. Healthcare systems, academic medical centers, private equity-backed groups — they all benefit when physicians frame their own exploitation as devotion. You don't need to pay someone more if they believe their sacrifice is the point. You don't need to fix administrative burden if physicians absorb it as part of the calling. You don't need sustainable staffing models if the culture defines unsustainability as virtue.

The calling language does something more insidious too. It turns limits into failures. If you need to leave work at a reasonable hour to be home for dinner, that's not time management. In the vocation frame, it's a crack in your dedication. If you decline extra call, that's not a reasonable boundary. It's evidence that you weren't really cut out for this. If you're considering leaving medicine, that's not a legitimate career decision. It's abandonment.

This is how the vocation trap closes. You go in believing the calling is real, because it is. You absorb a culture that tells you sacrifice proves that calling. You start measuring your own worth by how much you're willing to give up. And when the giving becomes unsustainable, you don't blame the system. You blame yourself.

That's by design.

The "calling" frame isn't inherently wrong. Medicine can be both meaningful and fair. You can love what you do and still insist on being paid adequately, working sane hours, and maintaining a life outside the hospital. Those things aren't in conflict, unless someone needs them to be.

The toxic version of the calling culture is the one that treats suffering as proof of commitment. Any culture that responds to physician exhaustion with reminders about privilege isn't interested in your wellbeing. It's interested in your compliance.

The vocation trap is also self-sealing. The more deeply you've internalized the calling frame, the harder it is to question it from the inside. Questioning it starts to feel like questioning your own character, your own values, your own reasons for going into medicine in the first place. That's the trap. The system put those feelings there. They're real feelings, but they're also serving a function that has nothing to do with your wellbeing.

Notice the pattern in your own environment. Listen for moments when your legitimate needs get framed as entitlement. Watch for how the language of medicine's nobility gets used to justify institutional decisions that benefit the organization at your expense. When a struggling physician raises concerns about workload and the response is a reminder about patient trust, that's not a conversation about medicine's meaning. It's a way of shutting the conversation down.

The calling is real. The weaponization of it isn't something you need to accept.

Breaking the Spell

The first thing that breaks the spell is naming what it is.

Toxic calling culture is a management strategy. It may not be deliberately cynical in every case. Some people perpetuating it genuinely believe it. But regardless of intent, the effect is the same: physicians absorb conditions that damage them, and the institution pays no price for that damage.

Naming it doesn't require cynicism about medicine. You can still believe the work matters and recognize that the culture surrounding it has been shaped to extract more from you than you can sustainably give.

The second thing that breaks the spell is separating your identity from your endurance.

In the vocation frame, a good physician is one who endures. The physician who takes call without complaint, who absorbs the inbox without pushing back, who volunteers for every committee, who never says the system is broken — that's the model physician. The ones who set limits get quietly filed away as less committed.

Endurance is not the measure of clinical excellence. Your diagnostic skill doesn't improve because you're exhausted. Your patient relationships don't deepen because you haven't taken a real break in two years. Your ability to make good decisions doesn't sharpen when you're running on inadequate sleep and back-to-back double-booked clinic sessions.

The physician who maintains their capacity, who protects their focus and mental clarity, who has a life outside the hospital, is a better physician than the one who burns down trying to prove devotion. Separating identity from endurance means building a different answer to the question "What kind of doctor am I?" The answer doesn't have to involve martyrdom.

The third piece is understanding how academic hierarchies sustain the spell.

Academic medicine has a steep status ladder. Medical school prestige, residency reputation, fellowship pedigree, publishing record, grant funding, h-index — it's a layered hierarchy with its own currency. That hierarchy creates real stakes. People who've climbed it have strong reasons to defend the system that rewarded them. People still climbing it have strong reasons not to challenge it.

This is why dissent in academic medicine is so hard. Questioning the calling culture or the working conditions risks your reputation with the people who control your academic future. A junior faculty member who challenges the hidden contract takes a real professional risk. The culture knows this and uses it.

You don't have to be a martyr here, either. Breaking the spell doesn't require a public declaration. It starts with internal clarity.

Know what you believe about your own worth and your own limits, separate from what the culture has told you. Know the difference between feeling genuinely fulfilled by meaningful work and feeling trapped in suffering that's been rebranded as purpose. These feel different when you pay attention. One leaves you tired but replenished. The other leaves you depleted and vaguely ashamed of being depleted.

Find your people. Every academic department has physicians who've quietly decided to maintain their limits, who've chosen a different relationship with the hierarchy, who can see the pressure for what it is without blowing up their careers over it. These people are harder to spot because they don't announce themselves. They're usually the ones who leave on time, who decline extra committee work without visible guilt, who give honest answers when you ask how they're really doing.

Seek those people out. Not for permission, but for perspective. When you're surrounded only by people performing total devotion, it's easy to think that's the only way. It's not.

The last thing to understand is that leaving academic medicine, if that's where you land, isn't failure.

Academic medicine presents itself as the pinnacle. The culture implies that leaving for community practice or a non-clinical role is a step down, a retreat, a sign that you couldn't cut it. That framing is also a management tool. If you believe leaving is failure, you'll tolerate conditions that would otherwise be intolerable.

Community practice isn't a consolation prize. Direct primary care, hospitalist work, concierge medicine, locum tenens, non-clinical roles — none of these are lesser paths. Many physicians who leave academic medicine describe it as the first time they felt like a physician again, rather than an academic laborer. The prestige trade-off is real. So is the freedom.

If the ivory tower is where you want to be, fight for better conditions inside it. Build coalitions with other faculty. Document what's happening to your protected time. Push back formally when commitments get broken. The system doesn't repair itself, but it can be moved when enough people push in the same direction.

If the ivory tower is holding you in place because leaving feels like betrayal or failure, that's the spell talking.

What to Do With This Information

Three concrete moves from here.

Audit the calling language in your environment. For the next two weeks, pay attention to how your institution uses the language of medicine's meaning. Notice when patient care gets invoked not to make a clinical point but to justify an administrative demand. Notice when your own sense of calling gets turned against your own interests. You don't have to confront anyone yet. Just see it clearly.

Track your protected time reality. If you're in academic medicine with a research or administrative allocation, pull up what you were promised and document what you're actually getting over the next 30 days. Clinical time that eats into your protected allocation is unpaid labor. Knowing the gap is the first step to addressing it formally, whether that means a conversation with your chair, a renegotiated agreement, or a decision about where to take your career next.

Name your actual calling in your own words. Find one part of your practice that still gives you something real — a patient population, a procedure, a teaching relationship, a diagnostic challenge — and write down in a few sentences why it matters to you. Use your own language, not institutional language. That's the part of the calling that genuinely belongs to you. The rest is someone else's story about what you owe them. Keeping those two things separate is how you protect the real thing from being used against you.

The ivory tower was supposed to protect intellectual freedom. For a lot of physicians inside it today, it's become another kind of constraint, more refined than a corporate contract, more insidious because it's wrapped in language you actually believe in. You can see the structure clearly now. That changes what you can do about it.

The Gender Attrition Gap

Women now make up roughly half of all medical school graduates in the United States. They entered the pipeline in record numbers. They matched, completed residency, passed boards, and joined practices. And then, at a rate 43% higher than their male colleagues, they left.

That's what the hazard ratio of 1.43 means. Female physicians are 43% more likely to exit clinical medicine than male physicians. And they're doing it younger. The median exit age for women is 49. For men, it's 64. That's not a small gap. That's 15 years of clinical career cut short, consistently, across the profession.

The system calls this a "pipeline problem." It blames women's choices: family, balance, preference. It frames early exit as a personal decision. What it doesn't say is that the profession was never actually built to retain them.

This chapter is about what's really happening, why the structural failures run deeper than most institutions will admit, and what female physicians can do right now to protect themselves in a system still designed around someone else.

The Data on Female Physician Exit

A hazard ratio of 1.43 is not a rounding error. In epidemiology terms, that's a strong signal. It means if you follow two equally qualified cohorts of physicians into practice, one male and one female, you can predict with confidence that the women will leave at substantially higher rates and substantially earlier. The profession has known this pattern for years. It hasn't fixed it.

The median exit age data tells an equally clear story. When women leave at 49 and men leave at 64, you're looking at a profession that's burning through its female workforce in the middle of their peak earning and peak experience years. These aren't physicians at the end of long careers deciding it's time to retire. These are physicians in their late 40s making the calculation that staying isn't worth what it costs.

That calculation is rational. When you look at what female physicians are asked to absorb relative to their male peers, the surprise isn't that women leave. The surprise is that so many stay as long as they do.

The gender pay gap in medicine is real and documented. Female physicians earn less than male physicians across specialties, even after controlling for hours worked and patient volume. The gap compounds over time. A female physician earning less per year for 20 years loses hundreds of thousands of dollars in cumulative income. That affects retirement savings, loan payoff timelines, and financial runway in ways that don't show up in any wellness survey.

The leadership gap follows the same pattern. Women are underrepresented in department chair positions, in C-suite roles at health systems, in specialty society leadership, and on the committees that actually set policy. This matters because the people who design physician work environments are disproportionately male. They're designing for their own experience, which is not the same experience female physicians are having.

The Structural Failures

The standard framing is that women in medicine struggle with "work-life balance." That phrase does a lot of work to obscure what's actually happening. It implies the problem is personal time management. It suggests that if a female physician could just optimize her schedule better, everything would be fine.

The structural failures are different. They're baked into how medicine is organized.

Parental leave policies in many healthcare systems remain inadequate or inconsistently applied. Some institutions offer robust leave; many don't. Residents and fellows are often particularly unprotected, completing training during exactly the years when many women are building families. Pregnancy during residency isn't a crisis to plan for. It should be a normal life event that the system accommodates. In many programs, it still isn't.

Childcare infrastructure at hospitals is rare. Most physicians, regardless of gender, manage childcare on their own. But the burden falls disproportionately on female physicians in dual-physician households and in single-parent situations. When a child is sick and someone needs to leave, the cultural expectation of who that someone is doesn't fall equally.

On-call schedules weren't designed with primary caregivers in mind. That's not a conspiracy. It's a legacy of designing the physician workforce as if physicians had a spouse at home managing everything else. Many male physicians historically did. Many female physicians don't have that same setup.

Breastfeeding accommodations are legally required in many settings but practically difficult to access when you're booked solid and your patients are waiting. A 20-minute window between patients that barely exists for a bathroom break certainly doesn't accommodate pumping. The physician who tries to manage this is navigating a structural failure every single day while also being expected to perform at full capacity.

These aren't minor inconveniences. Stacked together and sustained over years, they create a chronic drain that the profession then interprets as individual weakness or poor fit. It isn't weakness. It's a rational response to a system that extracts full performance while providing inadequate support.

Compounding Disadvantages

The pay gap, the leadership gap, and the caregiving burden don't exist in isolation. They compound.

A female physician earning less than her male peer has less financial cushion when she needs it. She has less ability to tolerate a bad employment situation. She has less leverage in contract negotiations because her runway is shorter. Her golden handcuffs feel tighter, even if the dollar amounts are smaller, because the gap between what she earns and what she'd need to feel financially secure is wider.

The leadership gap compounds too. When women aren't in the rooms where decisions get made, the decisions reflect that absence. Scheduling policies, parental leave structures, call distribution, and administrative burdens don't get redesigned because the people doing the redesigning aren't experiencing them the same way. Women who do reach leadership positions often find themselves carrying an additional weight: expected to fix the systemic problems while also performing the same job they were hired to do.

The invisible labor gap sits underneath all of it. Research across industries consistently shows that women absorb more unpaid organizational labor than men: mentoring junior colleagues, serving on diversity committees, managing interpersonal conflicts on their teams, performing the emotional labor that keeps a unit functioning. Medicine is no different. A female attending who mentors four medical students, chairs the wellness committee, and mediates the tension between the nurses and the new resident is doing work that doesn't count in any RVU calculation and doesn't appear in any performance review.

She's also probably doing more at home.

The double shift, paid work plus the majority of household and caregiving labor, is a documented pattern in dual-income households. Physicians are not immune to it. A female physician who finishes a 10-hour clinical day, drives home, handles the domestic evening routine, and then sits down for two more hours of inbox management is not burning out because of personal weakness. She's burning out because she's working two full-time jobs simultaneously and her profession is only counting one of them.

The harassment and gender bias layer compounds everything further. Female physicians report being mistaken for nurses at rates their male colleagues don't experience. They're called by their first name by staff and patients while their male colleagues are addressed as "Doctor." Their clinical authority is questioned at rates that don't match their credentials. They receive feedback on their communication style that amounts to being told they're either too assertive or not assertive enough, depending on who's doing the evaluating.

None of this is the primary driver of the 1.43 hazard ratio by itself. But none of it disappears either. It accumulates in the background of every clinical day until the calculus shifts.

What Must Change, and What Physicians Can Do Now

The systemic changes need to happen at the institutional level, at the specialty society level, at the legislative level. More on collective action in Chapter 15. Right now, this section is about what you can actually control.

Know your numbers. If you don't know what your male colleagues in equivalent roles are being paid, find out. Many states now have pay transparency laws. Specialty societies publish compensation data. Ask directly when you're in a position to ask. You can't negotiate the gap you can't see.

Document the invisible labor. Keep a running log of every committee you sit on, every mentorship conversation you conduct, every organizational task you absorb that isn't in your job description. This documentation serves two purposes. First, it gives you concrete evidence when you ask for compensation adjustments, schedule accommodations, or role modifications. Second, it makes visible to you how much you're actually carrying. Many physicians who feel vaguely exhausted haven't totaled the weight. When you see it written down, you can decide what to renegotiate.

Read your contract with gender-specific questions. Chapter 9 covers contract anatomy in detail. For this chapter, the specific question is: what does your contract say about parental leave, call coverage during leave, return-to-work ramp-up, and part-time arrangements? Many contracts are silent on all of these. Silent means the institution decides. That's not a position you want to be in when you actually need it.

If your contract is silent on parental leave specifics, ask for language before you sign. Get it in writing. "We'll work something out" is not a contractual commitment.

Build your clinical peer network deliberately. Female physicians who leave clinical medicine often cite isolation as a significant factor. When you're the only woman in a practice, or one of two, you absorb the full weight of being a representative while also managing your own caseload. A deliberate peer network, physicians outside your institution who you can talk to honestly, changes the calculus. You need people who've navigated similar situations and can tell you what's actually possible.

Set boundaries on organizational labor. This is covered in depth in Chapter 11, but the gender-specific application is this: if you're being asked to serve on more committees than your male peers, you're allowed to say no. If you're the de facto emotional support for your entire unit, you're allowed to redirect. The willingness to take on this labor is a strength. Being exploited for that willingness is a structural problem you don't have to absorb individually.

Consider schedule modification as a financial and career decision. Some female physicians who feel the pull to leave clinical medicine entirely would actually thrive in a modified role. This might mean reducing from full-time to four days per week. It might mean transitioning to a DPC or concierge model that gives more schedule control. It might mean cutting administrative committees entirely and protecting pure clinical time. The triage model in Chapter 14 walks through how to make this assessment systematically. The point here is that the option between "stay exactly as I am" and "leave entirely" isn't binary.

Know what the early exit data means for your retirement math. A female physician who exits at 49 instead of 64 has 15 fewer earning years. That affects retirement savings, Social Security calculations, and financial independence timelines. If you're considering leaving clinical medicine, Chapter 13's Runway Number calculation is especially important. You need to know exactly what your financial position looks like before you make the move, not after.

Don't absorb the institutional gaslighting. You've heard it. "Women just choose different lifestyles." "You need to be more resilient." "Medicine is hard for everyone." These framings put the responsibility for a structural problem onto the individuals it's harming. The hazard ratio of 1.43 isn't a lifestyle choice. The 15-year gap in median exit age isn't explained by preference. If you've internalized any part of the narrative that your exhaustion is your own failure, this chapter exists to offer a correction.

The system is failing female physicians at scale. That's a verifiable fact, and you're not obligated to pretend otherwise.

The Attrition Is a System Problem, Not a Personal One

There's a version of this chapter that ends with reassurance. You're strong. You can do this. Medicine needs you.

That version of the chapter would be lying to you.

Medicine does need you. That's also true. But "medicine needs you" is not a sustainable reason to stay in a role that's destroying your health, your financial security, and your sense of self. It's a version of the calling argument that Chapter 7 already dismantled. The profession doesn't get to extract you and then ask you to stay for the good of the cause.

Female physicians are leaving 15 years earlier than their male counterparts. The structural reasons for that are real. The failure to fix those structures is a choice that healthcare institutions are making, whether consciously or by inertia. You didn't create that situation and you can't fix it by working harder.

What you can do is make a clear-eyed decision about your own path forward. The tools to do that are in this book. The Four-Path Triage Model in Chapter 14 applies to every physician in this situation, regardless of gender. The financial sovereignty framework in Chapter 13 applies equally. The boundary scripts and contract checklists don't have a gender requirement.

What this chapter adds is the specific framing that female physicians often need to hear: your exhaustion makes complete sense given what you're carrying. The data confirms it. The structure created it. Your choice, whatever it is, deserves to be made based on what you actually need, not on what the system has decided you should be able to tolerate.

Your Next Move

Three specific actions before you move to the next chapter.

First, pull your most recent compensation data and compare it against the specialty benchmark for your role, your geography, and your experience level. If you don't know where to find that data, your specialty society publishes it. If you're below market, that information belongs in your next contract conversation.

Second, spend 15 minutes listing every piece of organizational labor you're doing that isn't in your job description. Don't filter. Don't minimize. Just list it. Then look at the list and identify one item you're going to stop doing or delegate in the next 30 days. One item. That's the starting point.

Third, check your contract for parental leave, call coverage, and part-time provisions. If those sections don't exist or are vague, flag them before you need them. The time to negotiate those terms is before they're urgent, not during.

The system's failure to retain female physicians at the rates it should is a documented fact. What you do with that information is still your call.

The Contract, the RVU, and the Golden Handcuffs

The signing bonus check arrives, and it feels like validation. After years of training, debt accumulation, and deferred life, someone is finally paying you what you're worth. Or so it seems.

Most physicians sign their first employment contract without a healthcare attorney. They skim the compensation section, note the base salary and bonus structure, and initial every page. The rest feels like legal boilerplate, too dense to matter.

It does matter. Every clause matters.

The employment contract is the document that determines whether you have options or you're trapped. And by the time most physicians figure out the difference, they've already signed.

Anatomy of a Predatory Contract

A predatory physician employment contract doesn't announce itself. It looks like every other contract you've seen, which isn't many, because residency doesn't teach contract law. It uses standard formatting, professional language, and a generous-sounding compensation package on page one. The traps are buried in sections most physicians skip.

The noncompete clause is the most common. It restricts where you can practice if you leave, usually within a geographic radius and for a set period of time. A 25-mile radius and a two-year restriction might sound reasonable until you realize your entire referral network, patient population, and professional identity are inside that circle. Leaving the job means leaving the region or starting from scratch.

Noncompete enforceability varies by state. Some states, including California, have largely prohibited them for physicians. Others enforce them aggressively. Many physicians don't find out which category their state falls into until they're trying to leave and receive a cease-and-desist letter from their former employer's legal team.

Tail coverage is the second trap. Malpractice insurance comes in two forms: occurrence-based, which covers claims from events that happened during your employment period regardless of when you leave, and claims-made, which only covers claims filed while you're still employed. Most employers use claims-made policies because they're cheaper. The "tail" is the extension you need after leaving to stay covered for anything that happened while you were there.

Tail coverage can cost tens of thousands of dollars. Who pays it matters enormously. Many contracts place the full tail burden on the departing physician. That means leaving the job triggers a five-figure expense on top of the income disruption of starting somewhere new. It's a financial disincentive to exit, built directly into the contract.

Then there's the termination clause. Contracts often give the employer the right to terminate "without cause" with 60 to 90 days' notice. You can be let go for any reason, or no stated reason at all. The physician's ability to leave on the same terms is often more restricted, requiring longer notice periods tied to noncompete and tail-coverage obligations that activate the moment you walk out.

On-call requirements and APP oversight expectations frequently appear buried in addendums rather than the main contract body. You might sign what looks like a reasonable practice agreement and only later discover you're expected to supervise a panel of advanced practice providers whose charts you're legally responsible for, or that you're on call every third weekend with no cap on consult volume.

Read every addendum. Read every exhibit. Read the employee handbook that the contract incorporates by reference, because if the contract says the handbook governs your conduct and the handbook can be changed at will by your employer, they can rewrite the rules without your signature.

The RVU Trap

Relative Value Units were designed by Medicare as a standardized way to measure physician work and reimburse accordingly. The theory had some logic: assign a unit value to each service based on the time, skill, and complexity it requires, then pay based on how many units a physician produces. In practice, the RVU system became the architecture for an assembly line.

Your compensation is tied to a productivity formula you didn't negotiate and can't meaningfully control. The payer mix in your panel affects your effective rate. The administrative tasks attached to each visit consume time without generating units. The prior authorizations, the inbox messages, the care coordination calls: none of that generates RVUs. You do the work. The meter doesn't move.

RVU benchmarks are typically drawn from national survey data, and many employers set targets at or above the 50th or 75th percentile of physician productivity. This sounds fair until you realize the benchmark is a moving target. As more physicians grind harder under productivity pressure, the average rises. Staying at the 75th percentile means working harder each year just to hold the same bonus threshold.

It's a treadmill that speeds up automatically.

Many contracts include a base salary that looks solid but only holds if you hit a minimum RVU threshold. Fall below it because you took FMLA, because your panel shrank, or because your health system reduced your clinic days, and your base pay gets clawed back. The compensation that felt like a floor turns out to have a trapdoor beneath it.

Overhead deductions can also erode your effective rate dramatically. Some contracts, particularly in private practice acquisitions by private equity groups, calculate physician compensation after deducting overhead as a percentage of collections. If overhead costs rise because management added administrative layers, remodeled the facility, or changed the EMR vendor, those costs come out of your paycheck. You had no vote on any of those decisions.

You're a partner in name, an employee in practice, and a line item in a spreadsheet in reality.

The RVU model creates a quiet pressure to see more volume. More visits per day means more units. But more volume per physician means less time per patient, more documentation shortcuts, more follow-up inbox volume the next morning, and more room for error. The system rewards throughput and treats physician wellbeing as a rounding error.

Some contracts include quality bonuses layered on top of RVU productivity, tied to patient satisfaction scores, HEDIS metrics, or value-based care outcomes. These sound reasonable on paper. Patient satisfaction scores are influenced by factors outside your control, including wait times set by scheduling staff, parking lot availability, and whether you declined to prescribe something a patient wanted. Tying your income to scores that measure things you can't control is just another way to put your pay at risk.

Post-Residency Overleveraging

The financial context in which most physicians sign their first contract is worth stating directly. The average medical school graduate carries significant debt. Residency salaries rarely cover more than living expenses in high-cost cities. By the time a physician reaches their first attending position, they've been in school and training for over a decade, with net worth deeply in the negative.

Into that financial reality walks a recruiter with a signing bonus, a relocation package, a salary that looks enormous compared to residency pay, and a contract that needs to be signed before the offer expires.

The pressure to sign quickly is often real and sometimes manufactured. Offers do expire. Good positions do get filled. But urgency framing also serves the employer. A physician who takes six weeks to have the contract reviewed by a healthcare attorney is a physician who might negotiate or walk away. Speed works in the employer's favor.

Post-residency overleveraging typically unfolds like this: the physician signs the contract, accepts the signing bonus, uses the relocation package, buys or leases a home based on the new income, and starts building a life in a new location. Within six to twelve months, the problems buried in the contract begin surfacing in daily work. The call schedule is heavier than expected. The RVU targets are harder to hit than the recruiter implied. The management culture is exactly what the last round of departing residents warned about.

But now you've spent the signing bonus. You're in a lease or a mortgage. Your noncompete covers your entire professional geography. Your tail coverage will cost you if you leave before the employer pays it out. Your student loans are in a repayment plan built around your current income.

You're not trapped by the walls. You're trapped by the paperwork.

This is overleveraging. A structural trap the system set, not a personal failure. And no one explained it in residency because contract negotiation isn't part of the medical education curriculum. The people who taught you to read a chest X-ray didn't teach you to read a clawback clause.

The clawback clause on signing bonuses deserves specific attention. Many physicians don't realize that if they leave within the specified period, they owe the full bonus back on a prorated schedule. A $50,000 signing bonus with a two-year clawback means leaving in year one could cost $25,000 out of pocket at exactly the moment your income is disrupted. Pair that with tail coverage costs, and the financial barrier to leaving can exceed the average physician's liquid savings.

This is the math that keeps burned-out doctors in jobs they've already mentally quit.

The debt variable compounds everything. Physicians carrying large student loan balances are often enrolled in income-driven repayment plans where monthly payments scale with earnings. Leaving a high-paying employed position doesn't just mean losing that income. It can mean losing the repayment trajectory, the Public Service Loan Forgiveness clock if they're in a qualifying position, and the financial stability the loan servicer built their current plan around. The economic exit cost isn't just the tail and the clawback. It's the entire financial architecture that was built around staying.

Employers know this. It isn't an accident that contracts are structured the way they are. The overleveraging isn't a side effect of a complicated hiring process. It's a feature.

The Contract Red Flag Checklist

You can't undo a contract you've already signed. But if you're on the front end of a job transition, or if you're trying to understand the actual leverage you have in your current role, working through these provisions gives you a clear map.

If you're reviewing a new offer, take it to a healthcare employment attorney before signing. Many attorneys who specialize in physician contracts charge a flat review fee that is a fraction of what a problematic contract will cost you over time in lost income, tail coverage, or clawback repayment. The fee is not optional overhead. It's the price of informed consent.

Noncompete provisions. Find the geographic radius and the time restriction. Map that radius against your actual practice location. Identify which patients, referral sources, and facilities fall inside it. Ask your attorney what the enforceability standard is in your state and whether any recent legislative or regulatory changes have affected noncompete law for physicians. If the employer won't move on the radius or duration, that refusal tells you something about how they view physician departure.

Tail coverage responsibility. The contract should specify who pays for tail coverage on departure. If it places the full burden on the departing physician, negotiate for shared responsibility or a sliding-scale employer contribution based on years of service. If the employer won't move on this at all, calculate the projected tail cost and factor it into your total compensation picture so you're making an informed decision, not a surprised one.

Termination clauses. Compare the employer's without-cause termination rights to your own exit rights. If your employer can let you go on 60 days' notice but you're required to give 90 days' notice and remain fully employed through that window, you're in an asymmetric arrangement. Confirm whether termination triggers your noncompete and tail-coverage obligations immediately or after a defined transition period.

Call schedule and coverage expectations. Don't rely on anything a recruiter says verbally. The contract or its addendums should specify call frequency, how unplanned coverage gaps are handled, and whether there's any cap on consult volume during call periods. Vague language here is a warning sign. Push for specifics in writing before you sign.

APP oversight obligations. Many contracts now include supervisory responsibility for advanced practice providers as a condition of employment, sometimes with legal liability attached, and without separate compensation. Identify whether you're expected to supervise APPs, how many, and what the legal supervision framework is in your state. Know this before you agree to it.

RVU target and compensation floor. Read the base salary guarantee carefully. Identify what happens if you fall below the minimum productivity threshold. Check whether your contract converts to a pure RVU model after a guarantee period ends, what the effective conversion rate would be, and how overhead is calculated if you're in a collections-based model. Run the math on what your compensation would look like in year three versus year one.

Signing bonus clawback terms. Identify the repayment period and the proration schedule. Do the math on what leaving in year one versus year two would actually cost you in dollars. Factor that number against your projected savings during the guarantee period. If the clawback exposure is higher than your liquid savings, that's a constraint worth knowing before it's a crisis.

Dispute resolution terms. Some contracts require binding arbitration for all disputes, waiving your right to a jury trial. The arbitration venue and governing law provisions matter if you're practicing in a different state than where the corporate parent is headquartered.

Change-of-control provisions. If your employer is acquired by another health system or a private equity group, what happens to your contract? Some contracts include automatic assignment clauses that transfer your employment to the acquiring entity without requiring your consent. Others give you termination rights. Acquisitions in healthcare are not rare. Know which category your contract falls into before any rumor of a deal starts circulating.

Income guarantee timing. If your contract includes an income guarantee for the first year or two, verify the exact end date and what the conversion looks like when it expires. Some physicians discover the hard way that their guarantee ended earlier than they remembered, or that the productivity model it converts to pays significantly less than their current effective rate.

This checklist doesn't replace a healthcare attorney. Use it as preparation so your attorney review is focused, efficient, and specific.

What Leverage Actually Looks Like

Physician employment contracts are negotiable, even when employers act as though they aren't.

Health systems and private practices prefer standardized agreements because standardization reduces their administrative burden. When a physician pushes back, the default response is often to say the contract is non-negotiable, that everyone signs the same form. This is sometimes true. Frequently it isn't.

Physicians who win concessions are the ones who've done the homework, who know exactly what they're asking for, who negotiate through an attorney rather than in a face-to-face conversation where social pressure narrows options, and who are genuinely prepared to walk away from a deal that doesn't meet minimum standards.

Walking away requires having an alternative. That's the core of the golden handcuffs problem. When you have no financial runway, no other offer in progress, and no negotiated exit path, you sign what's in front of you. Chapter 13 addresses financial sovereignty and building that runway in detail. For now, the basic point is that a contract signed under financial pressure, inside a short window, without legal review, while carrying six-figure debt, is a contract that was designed to be signed exactly that way.

The urgency, the complexity, the length, the buried addendums, the recruiter who seems to be on your side but works for the employer: these are features working together.

Your degree took a decade to earn. The contract you sign with it deserves more than a weekend read.

Three Things to Do Now

1. If you're currently employed and haven't read your contract recently, read it this week. Pull the original document, including every addendum and exhibit. Focus on

the termination rights, noncompete geography, tail coverage responsibility, and the RVU floor attached to your base salary. Flag every clause you don't understand, then take those specific questions to a healthcare employment attorney.

1. If you're evaluating a new offer, budget for an attorney review before signing. Search specifically for attorneys who specialize in physician employment contracts, not general employment law. The specialty matters because tail coverage structures, RVU compensation models, and APP oversight liability have nuances that general practitioners routinely miss.

1. Calculate your clawback exposure today. If you accepted a signing bonus, find the clause and work out what you'd owe right now based on the proration schedule. This number is part of your financial reality whether or not you're planning to leave. Knowing it gives you information. Not knowing it gives someone else an advantage.

When the Doctor Breaks, Patients Lose Too

There's a conversation happening in hospital boardrooms and healthcare consulting firms that never quite makes it to the doctor's lounge. It goes something like this: physician burnout is unfortunate, a human resources problem, something to address with a wellness committee and maybe a gratitude journal initiative. Keep the doctors productive. Keep the RVUs flowing. Worry about morale later.

That framing is not just wrong. It's expensive. And for patients, it can be fatal.

Clinician wellbeing isn't a perk. It's a structural input to care quality the same way sterile instruments and functional imaging equipment are. When that input degrades, everything downstream degrades with it. Diagnosis quality. Communication. Error rates. Follow-through. Access. You already know this from your own worst shifts, the ones where exhaustion made you order a test you weren't sure you needed, or cut a patient conversation short, or miss a detail you'd normally catch. The system that created those shifts doesn't acknowledge what it costs the people on the other side of the exam room door.

This chapter names that cost directly. It also makes the business case healthcare administrators should be making but mostly aren't. And it gives you something useful: a frame for understanding that your wellbeing isn't a selfish concern. It's a public health issue. Claiming it is the most patient-centered thing you can do.

Clinician Wellness as a Patient Safety Metric

Burnout doesn't stay inside the doctor. It moves.

When a physician hits the depersonalization stage of the Maslach Triad, as we covered in Chapter 1, care delivery starts to change in measurable ways. Patients feel it first. The history is a little shorter. The explanation is a little thinner. The eye contact drops. The follow-up question doesn't get asked. These aren't failures of character. They're what happens when a human being has been running at or past capacity for months or years.

Research tracking burnout against clinical performance consistently shows that burned-out physicians have higher rates of medical errors, lower patient satisfaction scores, and reduced adherence to clinical guidelines. The relationship isn't subtle. Cognitive load, emotional depletion, and the cynicism that comes from sustained moral injury all compromise the mental bandwidth that medicine requires.

Medication errors go up. Near-misses increase. Preventable complications become more common. These outcomes don't show up on a physician's wellness survey. They show up in incident reports, malpractice filings, and patient harm events. By then, the connection to clinician wellbeing has been buried under layers of documentation and root cause analysis that almost never points at the burnout driving the system.

This is by design. The institutions profiting from physician labor have no incentive to establish a direct line between their productivity demands and patient harm. Naming that line is uncomfortable. It implies liability. It implies that the call schedule, the RVU target, the inbox volume, and the administrative burden weren't just hard on doctors. They were hard on patients.

The safety literature has been building this case for years. Patient safety researchers have documented the correlation between physician fatigue and error rates. Studies on resident work hours, ICU staffing ratios, and surgeon performance after night call all point the same direction: a tired, overwhelmed clinician is a risk factor. The profession has largely accepted this when it comes to sleep deprivation in trainees. It has been much slower to apply the same logic to the sustained, chronic depletion that defines attending physician burnout.

The gap between what we know and what institutions do about it is one of the most telling signs of how little physician wellbeing actually registers as a patient safety priority.

Access Erosion

When a burned-out physician leaves, a waiting room doesn't get cleared. It gets longer.

Physician shortages are already a defining feature of American healthcare in 2026, and they're getting worse. Primary care access is constrained in rural areas, in underserved urban neighborhoods, in specialties that have become too administratively burdened to attract new graduates. When an existing physician in one of those communities hits the wall and walks away, the patients they were serving don't disappear. They fall into the gap.

Some of them show up in emergency departments. Some of them delay care until a manageable problem becomes a crisis. Some of them drive an hour each way to see a provider who's also stretched too thin. Some of them don't get care at all.

The downstream effects of access erosion compound quickly. A diabetic patient who can't get a timely appointment loses glycemic control. A hypertensive patient who loses their primary care physician misses medication adjustments. A patient with vague chest discomfort who can't get in for three months waits until the symptom forces an ER visit. These outcomes are more expensive, more dangerous, and more preventable than anything a wellness retreat could fix.

The access problem isn't distributed evenly. Physicians who leave tend to leave markets that are already underserved. Rural communities, safety net hospitals, high-Medicaid practices, and specialties with brutal call requirements all lose doctors at higher rates. The patients those doctors leave behind have the fewest alternatives. They don't have the option to book a concierge practice or fly somewhere for specialty care. They absorb the loss directly.

This is worth sitting with if you're considering leaving clinical medicine. The question of whether to stay or go is ultimately yours to answer, and Chapter 14 will walk through that decision systematically. But the access reality is part of the honest picture. Your exit doesn't just affect your paycheck. It affects a panel of patients, some of whom have no backup option. That's not a guilt trip. It's context. It belongs in the calculation.

The system that burned you out created this shortage. It drove away the doctors before you. It's driving away your colleagues right now. The solution isn't to sacrifice yourself to a broken structure. The solution is to understand the stakes clearly and make your decision with clear eyes.

The Business Case for Physician Wellbeing

Healthcare administrators respond to numbers. So let's give them numbers.

Physician turnover is one of the most expensive operational failures in healthcare. When a physician leaves, the organization that employed them faces recruiting costs, credentialing timelines, productivity gaps during the search, locum coverage, and onboarding overhead for whoever eventually fills the role. Across the industry, estimates of total physician replacement cost run into the hundreds of thousands of dollars per position, with some specialty positions costing significantly more once lost productivity and coverage gaps are factored in.

That number sits next to the cost of wellness programming, flexible scheduling, inbox reform, and administrative support that could have prevented the exit. In almost every case, the prevention is cheaper. By a lot.

The math isn't complicated. Health systems often spend less than a thousand dollars per physician per year on wellbeing initiatives while facing turnover costs that can exceed half a million dollars per lost physician. If even one exit per year is prevented by meaningful wellbeing investment, the return is enormous. If administrators were running the same cost-benefit logic on any other operational input, they'd have solved this years ago.

They haven't solved it. The reasons are structural and worth naming.

First, turnover costs are distributed across departments. Recruiting sits in HR. Locum costs show up in staffing budgets. Lost productivity shows up in revenue shortfalls. Nobody builds a single line item that totals the full cost of losing a physician, so nobody feels the full weight of it in one place.

Second, wellness initiatives are treated as overhead. They appear on the expense side of the ledger without a corresponding revenue line. CFOs and COOs don't have a clean mechanism for crediting prevented turnover against the cost of an employee assistance program or a reduced-panel policy.

Third, and most honestly, physician wellbeing has historically been treated as a physician problem. Doctors are expected to absorb their own suffering. The idea that an organization has financial responsibility for the conditions that produce burnout challenges a cultural assumption that's been in place for decades.

That assumption is cracking. Publicly traded health systems and large hospital networks are starting to face pressure from investors, regulators, and accreditation bodies to account for physician attrition rates. Some state legislatures have begun looking at hospital staffing ratios and administrative burden documentation. The Joint Commission and other accrediting bodies have increased attention to clinician wellbeing as a patient safety factor. The pressure is slow, and it's nowhere near proportionate to the scale of the problem, but it's building.

You can use this. If you're in a position to advocate internally, the business case is your sharpest tool. Bringing turnover cost analysis to a departmental meeting or a medical staff committee meeting lands differently than presenting a wellness survey result. Administrators who won't fund a meditation room will sometimes fund an inbox reduction pilot when they understand what a single physician departure costs in real dollars.

Why This Framing Matters for Your Decision

The point of naming these costs isn't to make you feel responsible for a system you didn't design. It's to remove the distortion that makes burnout feel like a personal failing.

The dominant narrative around physician burnout still positions it as a resilience problem. You're struggling because you're not coping well enough, not mindful enough, not grateful enough. The system frames your exhaustion as evidence of your inadequacy rather than evidence of its dysfunction.

This chapter's argument cuts through that directly. Your exhaustion has measurable consequences for patient safety. Your potential exit has measurable consequences for access. Your depletion is a clinical supply chain failure, and the organization benefiting from your labor bears responsibility for it.

That framing does two things.

It lets you stop blaming yourself. Burnout isn't a character flaw in a physician who cares too much. It's a predictable outcome of a system that extracts more than it returns. You've been carrying a load that was never sized for one person. The error rates, the compassion fatigue, the shortcuts you've had to take, none of those are who you are. They're what happens when a competent professional is systematically overloaded.

It also gives you grounds to demand better. If clinician wellbeing is a patient safety issue, and the evidence says it is, then institutions have a safety obligation to address it. Prior authorization burdens that consume hours of clinical time per week are a patient safety issue. Inbox volumes that require two to three hours of uncompensated after-hours work are a patient safety issue. RVU targets that squeeze appointment slots to the point where history-taking is rushed are a patient safety issue. You're not asking for a vacation when you push back on these. You're asking for conditions that allow you to provide safe care.

Healthcare administrators have learned to use patient-centered language as a management tool. Patient satisfaction scores. Patient experience metrics. Patient-first culture. That language can be turned. If your institution genuinely means it, then clinician wellbeing belongs inside it. If they use the language without meaning it, pushing on that contradiction is still useful. It makes visible what the organization actually values, and that clarity is information you need.

This reframe also matters for colleagues, for medical staff meetings, for conversations with department chairs. "I can't keep doing this" sounds like a personal complaint. "Our current system creates patient safety risks, and here's the data" sounds like a professional concern. Same underlying reality, completely different institutional response.

What You Can Do With This

The argument that physician wellbeing is a patient safety issue is well-grounded, but it won't change your individual situation on its own. Here's where it becomes actionable.

Document your workload in safety terms. If you're seeing thirty-five patients per day when quality care requires twenty-two, that's a staffing ratio problem. If your inbox volume requires three hours of after-hours response time daily, that's an uncompensated labor problem with patient safety implications. Quantifying these conditions in writing, in terms that connect to care quality, creates a record that goes beyond personal complaint.

Track how your schedule affects care quality specifically. Note when appointments were too short to fully address a problem. Note when you had to defer a follow-up question because the schedule had already run over. Note when inbox backlog delayed a response to a patient concern. These notes are your evidence base. They're also useful if you ever need to make the case to a medical staff committee, a state medical board inquiry, or your own conscience.

Use the business case in institutional conversations. If you're part of a medical staff leadership structure, bring turnover cost data to conversations about workload and wellbeing investment. Most medical directors don't have this analysis ready-made. Presenting it reframes the conversation from "physicians are complaining" to "we have a retention and liability problem."

Look at what your institution's accreditation documentation says about physician wellbeing. The Joint Commission requires that organizations address clinician wellbeing as part of their safety programs. Many institutions have policy language that far exceeds their actual practice. That gap is a leverage point.

Stop accepting the resilience narrative. When wellness programming is offered as the response to structural problems, name the gap. "I appreciate the mindfulness session, but my inbox volume is still 120 messages per day, which means this isn't fixing the underlying problem." That sentence, delivered calmly and in writing, is more useful than either silent compliance or angry refusal.

If you're considering leaving clinical medicine entirely, take the access reality seriously without letting it trap you. The question to answer is whether staying in your current position serves your patients or whether a burned-out, demoralized version of you is actually the best clinical presence you can offer. Sometimes the most patient-centered decision is to step back, stabilize, and return in a role or structure that allows you to practice well. Sometimes it's to exit and create space for someone who hasn't yet been ground down.

The patients deserve a doctor who's functional. So do you.

The Gap Between What's Known and What's Done

It would be a short book if health systems were simply ignorant of the physician wellbeing data. They're not ignorant. The research is published in the same journals medical leadership reads. The turnover cost analyses are available from healthcare consulting firms that health systems already hire. The safety correlations have been in the literature long enough to have moved from emerging findings to established consensus.

What drives the gap between knowledge and action is incentive structure. Fee-for-service payment models reward volume. RVU-based compensation rewards throughput. Private equity ownership rewards margin compression. None of these incentive structures reward sustainable physician workloads. In fact, a physician who sets limits, leaves on time, and maintains a manageable panel is, from a purely financial optimization standpoint, underperforming.

The system was designed around physician self-sacrifice. Calling culture, as we covered in Chapter 7, elevated that sacrifice to a professional virtue. The corporate capture of medicine, as Chapter 6 laid out, then monetized it. The result is a structure that extracts maximum labor from physicians right up to the moment they quit or break, then replaces them at massive cost, and starts the cycle again.

Patients are the collateral damage in that cycle. They experience it as access problems, rushed appointments, communication gaps, and occasional errors. They don't have a way to connect those experiences to the working conditions of their physicians because the institutions controlling the narrative have every reason to keep that connection invisible.

Making it visible is part of what this chapter is for. And making it visible is part of what you can do, whether you stay and fight, modify your role, or eventually exit. The truth that physician depletion costs patients something real doesn't belong only in medical journals. It belongs in conversations with hospital administrators, in state legislatures considering healthcare workforce policy, in public discourse about what we actually want from a healthcare system.

You are not just a burned-out employee. You're a data point in a patient safety crisis that the people managing your labor have chosen not to fully acknowledge. That's worth knowing. It changes the shape of every conversation you're about to have.

Three actions to take now:

1. Quantify your own patient safety exposure. In writing, for one week, note the specific moments when your workload compressed the care you delivered. Rushed histories. Deferred follow-ups. Inbox delays. This isn't for guilt. It's for clarity and documentation.

1. Pull your institution's stated policy on clinician wellbeing. Most accredited organizations have language on file. Compare what the policy says to what your daily experience is. The gap between them is a formal lever, not just a personal grievance.

1. The next time a wellness initiative is offered as a response to a structural complaint, redirect it in writing. State the structural problem specifically, note that the offered response doesn't address it, and request a conversation about the structural fix. Keep a copy of your request.

The Power of No

You already know how to say no clinically. You say it dozens of times a week. No, that antibiotic isn't appropriate. No, this imaging isn't indicated. No, we're not doing that procedure because the risk outweighs the benefit. You say it with confidence because you've trained for it. You've got evidence behind you, years of clinical reasoning, and a professional obligation to the patient's wellbeing.

But the moment an administrator sends you a meeting invite for Saturday morning, the word vanishes. When a committee chair asks you to take on "just one more" project, you hear yourself saying you'll look into it. When the call schedule changes for the third time this quarter and your vacation gets swallowed up, you say nothing. You send a frustrated text to your spouse and show up anyway.

That gap — between clinical confidence and institutional passivity — is where burnout lives.

It's not a character flaw. It's a trained response. Medical culture spent the better part of a decade telling you that availability is professionalism, that sacrifice is virtue, and that a doctor who declines is a doctor who doesn't care enough. That message gets reinforced in residency, in attending evaluations, in the quiet social penalties you face when you're the first person to push back. By the time you reach mid-career, the pattern is so deeply wired that saying no to an unreasonable institutional demand feels physically uncomfortable.

This chapter is about rewiring that. Boundaries aren't a soft skill. They're clinical equipment. And learning to use them correctly is as important as any other tool you carry.

Boundaries as Medical Equipment

Think about sterile technique. Nobody frames it as a personality choice. Nobody asks whether you "feel comfortable" wearing gloves during a procedure. It's a standard that protects both the patient and the clinician. You don't negotiate it with administration. You don't soften it to avoid conflict. You do it because skipping it causes harm.

Boundaries work the same way. A physician without functional limits is operating without protection. The workload expands. The requests accumulate. The capacity to think clearly and care competently shrinks. And when that physician eventually breaks, the harm lands on patients, on colleagues who absorb the excess work, and on the physician's own health and career.

The framing matters. When you call a boundary a "personal preference," it sounds optional. When you understand it as a professional standard that protects your clinical capacity, it changes how you hold it, how you explain it, and how you respond when someone pushes back.

There's also a downstream reality worth naming. Every time you absorb a task that should have been declined, you signal that your time is available. Institutions aren't malicious in the way individuals can be malicious. They're opportunistic. They fill the space that exists. If your evenings are always available for inbox work, they'll keep scheduling things that require evening inbox work. If you always attend the optional committee meeting, it stops being optional. The pattern you establish becomes the expectation you inherit.

Saying no resets the pattern. It's a form of system communication, not just personal protection.

A Practical Inventory of What You Can Decline

Most physicians in employed or hospital settings have never actually reviewed what their contract obligates them to do versus what they do out of habit or social pressure. These are different categories, and the difference matters.

Here's a working inventory. Some of these will require contractual review. Others are purely cultural, meaning no document requires you to do them at all. Go through this list seriously.

Unpaid committee work. Most employed contracts specify clinical duties. Committee membership is often added informally, through an email invitation, a personal ask from a department chair, or a vague note in an onboarding packet. Unless your contract specifies committee participation as a job requirement, you're choosing to do this. You can decline or step back from committees that don't serve your patients or your career.

After-hours inbox responses. The expectation that patient messages sent at 9 p.m. deserve a response before midnight is a cultural norm, not a medical standard. Urgent clinical needs have established pathways: on-call lines, emergency departments, triage protocols. The portal message asking whether it's okay to take ibuprofen with a cold does not require a midnight response. You can set inbox hours. You can communicate them to patients. Practices that have done this report no meaningful increase in adverse events and a measurable reduction in physician after-hours labor.

Uncompensated administrative tasks. Prior authorizations, peer-to-peer reviews, appeal letters, prior approval renewals — these are labor. As covered in Chapter 2, the AMA documented that 44% of physicians report being unable to deliver necessary care because of prior authorization burdens. That work takes time. If it's not in your contract and it's not compensated, you have standing to raise that with administration. You may not win immediately, but documenting the time and raising it officially is a legitimate step.

Voluntary call beyond your contracted obligation. Call schedules are negotiated in contracts. If you're being pressured to cover shifts beyond your contractual obligation because of staffing shortages your employer created, that's a workforce management failure, not your personal responsibility. You can say no.

Mandatory "optional" meetings. If a meeting is truly optional, you can skip it. If attendance is actually required, it should be in your job description and compensated accordingly. Many institutions create a social penalty for non-attendance at meetings that are technically not required. That social pressure is real, but it's different from a contractual obligation. Know which category you're dealing with.

Scope creep outside your specialty. In under-resourced settings, physicians get asked to manage conditions outside their training because there's nobody else. This is a patient safety concern and a liability issue. You can and should decline tasks that fall outside your training and licensure scope, even when the institutional pressure to absorb them is significant.

Personal favors that erode professional time. Colleague requests for informal consultations, advice on their patients, review of their notes, or co-signature on forms they should be handling themselves all represent time. You can be collegial without being endlessly available. Saying "I can't take that on right now, let's schedule a formal consult" is a complete sentence.

This isn't an exhaustive list. The point is to distinguish what's obligated from what's habitual. Once you see that distinction clearly, you can make real choices about what to protect.

Boundary Scripts

Most physicians don't lack the desire to set limits. They lack the language. When you've spent years in a culture that equates availability with professionalism, it can feel like every decline needs a lengthy justification, an apology, or an elaborate explanation. It doesn't.

The scripts below are short and direct. They're designed to be used verbally or in writing. The goal is to be clear without being combative, and firm without leaving room for negotiation on the core point.

Declining a new committee or project:

"I appreciate you thinking of me. My current clinical load doesn't leave room for additional commitments right now. I'll have to pass."

You don't need to explain further. You don't need to suggest an alternative. You don't need to soften it with "but maybe next time." That's a complete decline.

Setting inbox hours:

"I respond to patient portal messages during scheduled administrative time, weekdays between [X] and [X]. Urgent needs should be directed to [triage line/on-call]. I'll get back to non-urgent messages within two business days."

This can go in your patient portal welcome message, your voicemail, and in writing to your practice manager. It sets an expectation before the problem occurs.

Declining after-hours administrative tasks:

"This is outside my compensated hours. I'll address it during my next scheduled admin block."

If a practice manager or supervisor assigns you after-hours work that isn't covered in your contract, this response is accurate and professional. You're not refusing to do the work. You're placing it where it belongs.

Peer-to-peer review calls outside working hours:

"I don't take peer-to-peer calls outside of [hours]. Please schedule through my office during those times."

Insurance companies and their review staff will often call at inconvenient times because availability works in their favor. It doesn't have to work in yours.

Pushing back on unilateral schedule changes:

"My contract specifies [X]. This change falls outside those terms. I need to review it with legal before agreeing."

You don't have to accept a schedule change verbally in the moment. You're allowed to take time, read your contract, and respond in writing.

Declining informal consultations:

"I want to be helpful, but I can't give you a reliable clinical opinion without seeing the patient through a formal consult. Let's set that up properly."

This protects you legally, protects the patient clinically, and puts the work where it belongs in the system.

Responding to guilt-based appeals:

"I understand the team is stretched. I'm not in a position to take on more right now."

Full stop. You don't need to explain your personal circumstances. You don't owe anyone a detailed accounting of why you're at capacity. "I'm not in a position to take on more right now" is a professional answer.

Notice what's not in any of these scripts: an apology. You're not sorry for having limits. You're not sorry for following your contract. You're not sorry for protecting your clinical focus. The apology has become so reflexive in physician culture that many doctors don't even notice they're doing it. Practice removing it. Watch how little changes when you do.

Anticipating and Holding Against Pushback

The first time you decline something you've always said yes to, you'll likely face pushback. That's predictable. Expect it and prepare for it.

Pushback comes in a few consistent forms, and each one has a clean response.

The guilt pivot. "If you can't cover, we'll have to cancel patients." This is an institutional staffing failure dressed up as your personal moral failing. When a system only functions if every individual absorbs unlimited demands, it's not a functional system. Your response: "I understand that's a challenge. I'm not available for this. The scheduling issue will need another solution." Then stop talking. Silence is not agreement. Silence is just silence.

The loyalty appeal. "We're a team here. We all have to pull together." This framing is designed to make your boundary sound like a betrayal of colleagues. But pulling together doesn't mean absorbing what an under-resourced system should be handling. Teams function on clear roles and sustainable workloads. Your response: "I'm committed to my contracted responsibilities. Taking on more than that isn't sustainable for me right now."

The minimizer. "It's just one meeting" or "It'll only take an hour." If it only takes an hour and it's so small, it shouldn't be hard for someone else to do it. Your response: "I know it sounds small, but I've got other commitments in that time. I can't add this."

The credential threat. "This could affect your performance review" or "People will notice." This is the most aggressive form of pushback, and it deserves the most careful handling. Document it in writing. If someone implies that declining a non-contractual obligation will harm your standing, that's a conversation worth having on the record. Your response in the moment: "I'd like to understand what my contracted obligations are in that area. Can we set up a meeting with HR to clarify?" That moves the conversation out of informal pressure and into accountable territory.

The emotional appeal. A colleague or supervisor who genuinely needs help, who's visibly struggling, who's asking you to cover because they're barely holding on themselves. This is the hardest. Your response here might be different from a corporate directive. You might choose to help this time. But be honest with yourself about the pattern. If you're consistently absorbing your own exhaustion plus someone else's because the system won't staff adequately, you're not being a good colleague. You're both drowning while the institution watches.

Holding a boundary under pressure requires one specific skill: the ability to let discomfort exist without acting to eliminate it. When someone pushes back and you feel the pull to cave, that discomfort is real. It's the old training activating. The instinct to smooth things over, to be accommodating, to prove you're a team player. You can feel that pull and still not move.

The practical tool is the broken record. You don't need new arguments. You don't need to win the debate or convince the other person you're right. You repeat the same position, calmly, without escalating. "I'm not able to take this on." Pause. "I understand you're in a tough spot. I'm not able to take this on." Pause. "I know this is frustrating. I'm not able to take this on." Three repetitions of a clear position, with no new justifications added, sends a message that the discussion is closed.

This isn't rudeness. It's clarity. And in a culture that thrives on physician ambiguity and deferred self-advocacy, clarity is a radical act.

What Saying No Does to the System

Individual boundaries don't fix broken institutions. That's important to say plainly. If your hospital has 30% APP oversight burden, if your EHR adds four hours of administrative work per physician per day, if your prior authorization queue runs 60 requests deep every Monday morning, your personal limit-setting doesn't eliminate those problems.

But it does something real. It shifts the burden back to the people responsible for fixing it.

When physicians consistently absorb institutional dysfunction without naming it or declining it, the system has no pressure to change. The problem stays invisible because the physicians keep solving it with their own time, health, and career longevity. When enough physicians decline to absorb the excess, the dysfunction becomes visible as a management problem, a staffing problem, a workflow problem. That's when it gets addressed.

You've already seen this in the data. The physician shortage driving so many of these pressures isn't a natural disaster. It's the predictable consequence of a system that grinds physicians down until they leave. Every physician who exits early removes capacity that costs millions to replace, if it can be replaced at all. Institutions that ignore physician burnout data are making a financial choice they'll eventually have to pay for. Your boundary, repeated by others, accelerates that reckoning.

There's also a modeling effect worth thinking about. If you're a department chair, a residency director, a senior attending, the culture you model becomes the culture the next generation absorbs. Every time you say yes when you should say no, in front of residents or junior colleagues, you're teaching them to do the same. Every time you hold a boundary professionally and calmly, you're showing them what's possible.

Your Next Move

This chapter gives you three specific actions to take before you move to the next one.

One: Run your own obligation audit. Pull out your employment contract and your most recent job description. Make two columns. Column one is what you're contractually required to do. Column two is what you're actually doing. Everything in column two that doesn't appear in column one is a choice. Some of those choices may be worth keeping. But you should be making them consciously, not by default.

Two: Draft your personal boundary script list. Go back through the scripts in this chapter and adapt them to your specific situation. Write down the three situations where you most often say yes when you'd rather say no. Write out the exact words you'll use the next time each one comes up. Practice them out loud. The discomfort of practicing in private is much smaller than the discomfort of freezing when it matters.

Three: Make one decline this week. A real one. Not a dramatic confrontation. Just one request you'd normally absorb that you instead respond to with a clean, professional no. Watch what happens. In most cases, the sky doesn't fall. The request gets routed somewhere else. The meeting proceeds without you. The committee finds another member. And you learn, through direct experience, that the consequences you feared were smaller than the cost of saying yes again.

That's where the shift starts. Not with a policy change or an administrative restructuring. It starts with one physician, in one moment, saying: I'm not available for that.

The word you already know how to say in the clinic. You just have to bring it out of the exam room.

Mental Health, Licensure Fear, and the Shame Machine

There's a specific kind of calculation physicians make when they're struggling. It goes something like this: if I tell anyone how bad it actually is, my license is at risk. My privileges could be pulled. My malpractice carrier might find out. My partners will question my judgment. My patients will lose confidence. So I'll handle it myself. I'll get through this week, and then next week will be better.

Next week is rarely better.

This calculation isn't irrational. It's the product of a system that spent decades treating physician mental health as a liability rather than a human reality. It's the product of credentialing applications that asked about past mental health care in ways that implied getting help was evidence of impairment. It's the product of a culture that celebrated stoicism, pathologized struggle, and trained you to believe that needing support meant you weren't cut out for the job.

The shame machine is real. It has moving parts, it runs continuously, and it's been running since your first year of medical school. Understanding how it works is the first step to getting out from under it.

The Architecture of Physician Shame

Physician culture is built on a particular story: that good doctors are resilient, that great doctors can absorb anything, and that struggling is a personal failing rather than a reasonable response to an unreasonable situation. This story gets layered in early.

In medical school, you learned to function on no sleep and call it training. You learned that showing stress was weakness and that weakness had professional consequences. You watched attendings perform certainty even when they didn't have it. You absorbed the lesson, even if nobody said it out loud. The job requires you to hold it together regardless of what's happening inside.

Residency deepens it. The hierarchy enforces it. The hours cement it. By the time you're an attending, the pattern is automatic. You manage what you're feeling so it doesn't show. You push through. You stay functional.

The problem isn't the ability to push through difficult moments. That's a genuinely useful skill. The problem is that the culture never gave you a clear signal about when to stop pushing and start getting help. The line between appropriate resilience and dangerous self-neglect got blurred, then erased entirely.

What fills the gap is shame. Shame says that asking for help is the same as admitting you can't do the job. Shame says that other people manage, so you should too. Shame says that disclosing your struggles to anyone creates a paper trail that could haunt you. And shame is incredibly effective at keeping people silent, isolated, and getting worse.

Physicians experience higher rates of depression and death by suicide than the general population. That's not a secret. What's less talked about is why the gap between suffering and getting help is so much wider for physicians than for almost anyone else. The barriers aren't just cultural. They're structural. They're baked into the very systems physicians interact with every day.

What Credentialing Questions Actually Ask

The single biggest barrier between physicians and mental health support isn't cost, time, or stigma, though all three matter. It's fear of what happens if it ends up on a credentialing application.

The fear is understandable. Physicians have seen colleagues lose hospital privileges, face board investigations, or have employment offers rescinded after disclosing mental health history. The concern isn't paranoid. It was historically well-founded.

But the landscape has shifted, and many physicians don't know it yet.

Credentialing questions vary significantly by state and by institution. For years, many applications asked broad, sweeping questions about mental health history: have you ever been treated for a mental health condition, have you ever seen a psychiatrist or counselor, do you have any history of emotional disturbance. These questions didn't distinguish between a physician who sought help briefly during a rough patch and one with an active, impairing condition. They treated any history of help-seeking as something to explain.

That design sent a clear message: getting care creates risk. And physicians responded accordingly by not getting care.

In recent years, a growing number of state medical boards have overhauled those questions after advocacy from physician wellness organizations, legal challenges, and federal guidance on disability discrimination law. The shift has been toward questions focused on current functional impairment rather than past treatment history. The key word is "currently." Many reformed applications now ask whether you currently have a condition that impairs your ability to practice medicine safely, rather than asking whether you've ever sought help for any mental health concern.

These are different questions with very different implications. Seeking support for burnout, stress, grief, or persistent low mood doesn't make you currently impaired. Working through something with a professional doesn't make you unfit to practice. A physician who got help, processed what needed processing, and returned to full function is not a liability. That's the framework that a reformed credentialing question reflects.

The catch is that reform isn't uniform. Some states have moved aggressively. Others haven't moved at all. Individual hospital credentialing committees have their own questions that may not reflect state board reforms. Insurance paneling applications can include their own disclosures. You need to know what specific questions apply to your specific situation before you make any decision about documentation.

That means reading your state board's current application carefully. It means looking at the exact language before you assume the worst. It means talking to a physician health attorney if you have real concerns about disclosure, because legal guidance in this area is far more affordable than the cost of staying sick to protect a license you're about to abandon anyway.

What you should not do is assume the worst-case scenario without checking the actual current rules. Physicians are trained to assess risk from evidence. Apply that same discipline here.

Navigating Physician Health Programs

Every state has a Physician Health Program, commonly called a PHP. These programs were created to help physicians with substance use disorders, but most have expanded to address a broader range of issues including burnout-related mental health struggles.

PHPs have a complicated reputation. Some operate as genuinely supportive, confidential programs designed to help physicians access care and return to healthy function. Others have a history of being punitive, invasive, and closely linked to state board reporting in ways that physicians found more threatening than helpful.

The variation matters. Before engaging with a PHP, it helps to understand how your state's program operates. Key questions include: Is participation confidential, and under what circumstances does the PHP report to the state board? What does monitoring look like? What are the exit criteria? Is participation voluntary or can it become mandatory?

Some states have made significant reforms to their PHPs in response to criticism. Advocacy groups representing physicians have pushed for programs that prioritize support over surveillance. The best PHPs function as a bridge between a struggling physician and appropriate care, with confidentiality protections that encourage people to reach out before a crisis forces intervention.

If you're uncertain about your state's PHP, talk to other physicians who've used it, or consult with a physician health attorney or your state medical society before making contact. Going in informed protects you. Going in blind can expose you to processes you didn't anticipate.

The existence of a PHP is not the same thing as the PHP being your only or best option. Many physicians get effective support entirely outside of PHP involvement, through private practitioners who specialize in working with healthcare professionals. These practitioners understand the unique pressures of medical culture, they understand credentialing realities, and they often structure their practice in ways that minimize documentation exposure.

State Board Reforms: Where Progress Is Happening

Reform is genuinely happening at the state board level, though it's uneven and still incomplete.

Several states have moved to what's called a "current impairment" standard, meaning their licensure questions focus only on whether a physician's condition currently affects their ability to practice safely. States that have adopted or moved toward this framework include some of the largest physician populations in the country. Medical associations in multiple states have lobbied successfully for language changes that protect physicians who proactively sought help.

The Federation of State Medical Boards has issued guidance recommending that boards move away from questions about mental health history and toward current functioning. That guidance doesn't bind individual state boards, but it signals which direction the professional consensus is moving.

There's also been meaningful action at the federal level. The Americans with Disabilities Act has been interpreted in ways that challenge overly broad mental health inquiries in professional licensing. Legal challenges have pushed some states to revise their applications. The argument, supported by disability rights law, is that blanket history questions about mental health treatment screen out people who sought help, which effectively penalizes proactive care-seeking behavior.

What this means practically is that the landscape in 2026 is substantially different from what it was ten years ago. A physician who avoided getting help in 2015 because of what they'd heard about licensure risk is operating on outdated information. That information gap is actively harming people.

The mental health stigma in medicine has always had two layers. The cultural layer, which is internal to the profession and is about shame and identity. And the structural layer, which is about what happens when help-seeking interacts with credentialing systems. Both layers are real. But the structural layer has weakened significantly in states where reform has taken hold, and it's worth knowing the current reality before making decisions based on the old one.

If your state hasn't reformed its questions yet, that's worth knowing too. It shapes how you approach confidentiality and what type of support makes sense given your specific risk picture.

The Specific Shame of High Performers

There's a particular version of the shame machine that targets high performers, and physicians are a concentrated population of high performers.

The logic goes: you've accomplished so much. You got through everything the system threw at you. People depend on you. Patients, colleagues, family. How could something be wrong with you? You should be grateful. You chose this. You're the one other people come to for help.

This version is especially effective because it weaponizes genuine strengths. The discipline that got you through training. The commitment to your patients. The sense of professional responsibility. It takes those real qualities and uses them as evidence that struggling is somehow incongruent with who you are.

It's not. Struggling is an entirely predictable response to working inside a system that's been documented, repeatedly, to break physicians. It's a reasonable response to moral injury, to inbox overload, to years of compounding pressure without adequate support. Feeling worn down under these conditions isn't a character flaw. It's a data point about your environment.

The high-performer version of shame is also connected to a specific fear: that getting help means admitting the career was a mistake. That if you couldn't handle it, maybe you weren't supposed to be here. This is a false conclusion drawn from a real feeling, and it's one of the most common things keeping physicians isolated.

Needing support doesn't mean you made the wrong choice. It means you've been carrying an extraordinary amount, often without adequate institutional backup, and that there are limits to what any person can sustain. Recognizing those limits isn't a failure. It's accurate self-assessment.

Finding Safe Help

"Safe" in this context means a few specific things. It means confidential within the limits that matter to you. It means competent for the specific situation you're in. And it means outside the institutional structures that have surveillance capacity over your career.

There are several categories of support worth knowing about.

Physicians who specialize in treating physicians. These practitioners understand the culture you work in. They know about the calling narrative, the shame architecture, the specific stresses of clinical medicine. They don't need you to spend sessions explaining why medicine is hard. They already know. Finding a practitioner with this background matters because it shortens the time to actually useful support and reduces the risk that the person you're talking to inadvertently minimizes what you're dealing with.

Employee Assistance Programs. Most hospitals and large group practices offer EAPs. They provide a limited number of sessions, often free. EAPs typically carry confidentiality protections that make them separate from your employer's records. If you've never explored what your institution's EAP actually offers, it's worth a look. For mild to moderate stress and pressure, a few focused sessions through an EAP can be a low-barrier starting point. For more significant situations, EAPs are usually a stepping stone rather than a complete solution.

Peer support programs. A growing number of hospitals have implemented peer support programs where trained physician peers offer a confidential space to talk after difficult cases, difficult stretches, or difficult decisions. These conversations are typically protected from disclosure and are explicitly designed not to create documentation. They're not a substitute for professional support when professional support is warranted, but they can break the isolation in the short term and open the door to more.

Private pay with private practitioners. Keeping mental health support entirely out of insurance records is possible when you pay privately. Many physicians choose this route specifically because it avoids the documentation trail that insurance billing creates. The cost is real, but for physicians close to their financial ceiling, the licensing protection tradeoff can make private pay the right call. Some practitioners offer sliding scale fees for exactly this population.

Online platforms with physician-specific programming. Several telehealth platforms have built offerings specifically for healthcare workers. These can be useful for physicians whose schedules make in-office appointments difficult and who want to start somewhere without a lot of friction. The confidentiality rules vary by platform, so it's worth reading the terms carefully.

One thing that matters across all of these categories: the quality of the match between you and the practitioner matters more than the category of service. A highly recommended provider who doesn't understand your specific professional context will be less useful than a lesser-known one who does. You're allowed to interview practitioners before committing. You're allowed to switch if the fit isn't working. Getting support isn't a one-shot decision where you have to accept whatever you find first.

The Practical Checklist Before You Reach Out

Before you make your first contact with any support provider, spend twenty minutes with these questions. The answers shape what kind of help you're looking for and how to approach it with appropriate care.

First, pull up your state medical board's current licensing application and find the mental health questions. Read the exact language. Note whether the questions refer to current impairment or historical treatment. If you're credentialed at a hospital, pull that application too. Know what you're working with before you assume the worst.

Second, if the language is broad or unclear, contact a physician health attorney for a one-hour consult. Not because you're in trouble, but because having a clear understanding of your actual legal landscape is a twenty-first-century professional responsibility. Many attorneys who specialize in physician licensing offer flat-fee consultations. Get information before you make decisions based on speculation.

Third, decide whether you want to go through your employer's EAP, a PHP, or a private practitioner. These aren't equivalent choices, and the right answer depends on your state's PHP structure, your insurance situation, your specific concerns, and your schedule. If you're uncertain, starting private and outside institutional structures is usually the more conservative choice.

Fourth, tell someone you trust. Not your department chair. Not your residency program director if you're still in training. Tell someone who isn't in a position of institutional authority over your career and who will help you stay accountable to actually following through. The gap between deciding to get help and actually showing up for it is where most physicians get stuck.

What Colleagues Get Wrong About This

When physicians talk to each other about mental health, two patterns tend to surface that are worth naming directly.

The first is competitive suffering. Someone mentions they're having a hard time, and the response is essentially: you think that's hard, wait until you hear what my week looked like. This isn't cruelty. It's a cultural reflex. But it forecloses the actual conversation and reinforces the idea that disclosing struggle makes you seem weak compared to colleagues who are managing.

The second is premature problem-solving. A colleague mentions struggling and within thirty seconds someone is recommending a mindfulness app, a weekend course on resilience, or a dietary change. The problem with premature problem-solving is that it skips the part where the struggling person feels heard. When you jump to solutions before someone has finished saying how bad it is, you send the message that you're uncomfortable with their distress and want to move past it quickly. That's not support. That's management.

If a colleague discloses that they're struggling, the most useful thing you can do first is stay with it. Ask what's been hardest. Don't pivot to solutions until they're ready. Normalize what they're experiencing without minimizing it. And mention, specifically, that the credentialing concerns they may have aren't necessarily what they think they are, and that it's worth getting accurate information before letting fear make the decision.

You can't fix the system for a colleague. But you can be the person who doesn't look away when they tell you the truth.

Your Next Move

The shame machine runs on isolation. The moment you start getting accurate information, it loses power. Here's where to start.

Check the actual language on your state board's current application. Not what you heard about it in residency. Not what a colleague told you ten years ago. The actual document, available on your state board's website right now. Knowing what the questions say is the single most important first step, because everything else depends on your real risk picture rather than the assumed one.

If you're currently struggling and haven't told anyone, tell someone this week. Not for accountability, not for advice. Just to break the isolation. A trusted colleague outside your direct institution, a spouse or partner, a friend who isn't in medicine. Say out loud what's actually been happening. The act of saying it makes the weight more manageable and makes the next step more possible.

If you're past the point where social support is enough, find a practitioner this week and schedule a first appointment before you lose the motivation. Not next month. This week. The appointment doesn't have to fix anything immediately. It just has to happen. The hardest part is the first session, and the first session starts with a phone call or a booking link.

Physicians are trained to catch problems early. You apply that standard to your patients every day. Apply it to yourself with the same rigor. The system won't do it for you. It's been demonstrated, repeatedly, that institutions prioritize your productivity over your wellbeing. That means this particular piece of your health is one you have to own.

Your license is worth protecting. So is your life.

Financial Sovereignty

Most physicians earn good money. Very few of them are free.

That gap between earning and freedom is where the system does some of its best work. You make a salary that looks impressive on paper. You take on a mortgage that matches it. You lease the car. You fund the private school tuition. You build a life that requires every dollar of your current income to stay intact. And then, when your hospital cuts your autonomy, loads your panel, or drops a performance improvement plan on your desk, you realize you can't leave. Not because there's nowhere to go. Because you can't afford the gap between now and there.

That's the golden handcuff, and it works precisely because it hides in plain sight. No one forced you into it. The system just made the choices that built it feel like normal adult behavior.

Financial sovereignty is what breaks that grip. It's the condition in which your ability to make a decision about your career does not depend on staying at your current job. It means having enough runway that you can say no to a bad contract, walk away from a toxic practice, or take six months to pivot without your credit cards absorbing the shock. It's not about being wealthy. It's about being free enough to choose.

This chapter is about building that freedom. Practically. Specifically. Starting now.

The Runway Number

The Runway Number is the single most clarifying piece of financial data you can calculate. It answers one question: how many months can you cover your essential expenses if your income stopped today?

That's it. One number. Months of freedom.

You're not calculating your net worth. You're not projecting retirement. You're calculating how long you can breathe without a paycheck before your life breaks down. That number tells you how much leverage you actually have.

Most physicians, when they run this calculation honestly for the first time, find that their Runway Number is somewhere between two and four months. That's it. Two to four months of freedom despite a decade-plus of high earning. That's not a personal failure. It's the predictable outcome of a lifestyle that expanded in lockstep with income, paired with a medical training culture that never taught financial strategy.

To calculate your Runway Number, you need two things. First, your true monthly essential expenses. Second, your current liquid assets.

Liquid assets means money you can access without a penalty and without selling something that takes weeks to settle. Cash in checking and savings accounts. A high-yield savings account. A money market fund. Investments in a taxable brokerage account that you could sell without a tax event that would cripple you. Your 401(k) or 403(b) does not count here unless you're close enough to retirement that early withdrawal penalties are negligible. Your home equity does not count unless you'd actually sell. Your car does not count.

Now divide your liquid assets by your essential monthly expenses. The result is your Runway Number in months.

If that number is under six, you're financially tethered to your current employer. They know it, even if they don't say it explicitly. A Runway Number under three means your employer holds almost all the leverage in every negotiation you have with them.

The goal is a Runway Number of twelve or more. Twelve months of free air. That's the point at which you genuinely have options. You can negotiate a contract from a position of strength. You can take the time to interview elsewhere without accepting the first offer out of desperation. You can launch a side income stream without panicking if it takes six months to ramp up.

Twelve months won't happen overnight. But every dollar you add to your liquid cushion increases your leverage. The direction matters as much as the destination.

Auditing Personal Overhead

You can't increase your Runway Number without knowing where your money is actually going. Most physicians skip this step because looking at the numbers feels like self-punishment. It's the opposite. Auditing your overhead is a power move. You're locating the places where your lifestyle is holding you hostage.

Start with fixed monthly obligations. Your mortgage or rent. Car payments. Insurance premiums. Private school tuition or childcare contracts. Minimum debt payments. Subscription services with annual commitments. These are the expenses that don't flex easily. Write them all down and get a total. This is your fixed monthly floor.

Then look at variable spending over the last three months. Pull your bank statements and credit card statements. Don't filter or judge yet. Just categorize. Dining and food. Travel. Clothing. Entertainment. Household services. Gifts. Professional memberships. Calculate a monthly average for each category.

Add fixed obligations to average variable spending. That's your current monthly burn rate.

Now separate that number into two columns. The first column is true essentials: housing, utilities, basic food, essential insurance, debt minimums, and childcare if it's required for you to work. The second column is lifestyle maintenance: everything else. Your Runway Number calculation uses only the first column, because in a genuine gap period, lifestyle maintenance is what you adjust.

The gap between your total monthly burn and your essential monthly expenses is your financial flexibility. If those two numbers are nearly identical, your lifestyle has no slack. If there's a significant gap, you have more runway than you think because the lifestyle column can compress in a crunch.

What you're looking for in this audit are the structural commitments that feel small but compound. The lease on a second vehicle that rarely gets driven. The high-end gym and the country club and the private concierge health service that together add up to more than a car payment. The restaurant and food delivery spending that, when honestly totaled, exceeds a mortgage payment. These aren't moral failures. They're data points. The question is whether each of those commitments is worth the career captivity it's buying you.

Physicians tend to carry specific overhead patterns worth flagging. Student loan payments, often at a minimum that doesn't attack principal aggressively, drain cash flow for decades without building any freedom-generating asset. A single home that's larger than needed can cost two to three times the equivalent in taxes, utilities, maintenance, and opportunity cost compared to a more modest one. And lifestyle inflation during residency and early attending years, the period when income spikes sharply, often locks in a burn rate that requires continuous high employment just to sustain.

None of this requires dramatic sacrifice. It requires a deliberate choice about which expenses are buying you something real and which ones are just the cost of keeping up with a social group that has the same golden handcuffs you're trying to break out of.

One practical approach: identify one or two overhead items totaling at least $1,500 per month that you could cut or defer for a defined twelve-month period. Direct that money straight to a liquid savings account earmarked as your runway fund. Don't invest it in something illiquid. Don't pay down a mortgage with it. Keep it accessible. Build the cushion first.

Why Physician Finances Are Structurally Different

The standard financial advice you'd find in a general money book doesn't fully account for what physicians face. The timing is different. The debt load is different. The income trajectory is inverted from most other high earners, meaning it starts very late and peaks at a point when most professions are already well into wealth accumulation.

A physician finishing training at thirty-two with $300,000 in student loans, entering a first contract under pressure to accept quickly, is structurally behind a peer who started earning at twenty-two even if the physician's income looks better on paper. The compounding gap from a decade of deferred earning is real.

Add the fact that many physician contracts include non-compete clauses that restrict where you can work if you leave. As covered in Chapter 9, those geographic restrictions can force a physician to either stay in a bad situation or uproot their family to exit. That's not a free labor market. It means the financial buffer you build has to be thick enough to absorb not just a gap in income but potentially a geographic transition cost.

And then there's the psychological piece. Physicians are socialized in training to defer personal needs. The culture punishes financial self-interest as somehow unseemly for someone in a healing profession. Asking for more money feels crass. Negotiating a contract feels aggressive. The result is a profession full of high earners who routinely accept below-market compensation, fail to negotiate signing bonuses or tail coverage, and don't build the financial structures that would give them real leverage.

Financial sovereignty isn't crass. It's what makes the rest of this book possible. You can't use the Four-Path Triage Model in Chapter 14 if every path except the status quo is financially impossible. Sovereignty is the precondition.

DPC and Concierge Models

For physicians who want to stay in clinical medicine but can't keep absorbing the corporate practice environment, Direct Primary Care and concierge medicine models represent a structural alternative worth understanding.

Direct Primary Care removes the insurance billing layer from primary care entirely. Patients pay a flat monthly membership fee, typically between $50 and $150 per month depending on the region and patient demographics. The physician keeps the fee, eliminates the billing department overhead, and carries a patient panel of around 400 to 600 patients instead of the 2,000-plus standard in insurance-based primary care. The administrative load drops substantially. The relationship with patients becomes more direct. Earnings are lower per hour on paper but higher per unit of sanity.

DPC doesn't work in every specialty. It's primarily a primary care and some specialty care model. But for the internists, family physicians, and general practitioners who make up a large share of the burnout statistics, it represents a genuine structural exit from the corporate production-line model described in Chapter 6.

The financial math matters. A DPC practice with 500 patients paying $100 per month generates $50,000 per month in gross revenue before overhead. A solo or small-group practice with modest overhead can yield a take-home that compares reasonably to an employed position, minus the RVU pressure, the administrator supervision, the inbox volume driven by a panel three times the size, and the sense that every clinical decision is being made for you.

Concierge medicine operates on a similar membership premise but at a higher price point. Annual fees ranging from $1,500 to over $10,000 per year are common, with practices carrying smaller panels of highly engaged patients who pay for guaranteed access and extended time. It skews toward markets with higher income demographics, but it's a real model that several thousand physicians currently run successfully.

Neither model is a magic fix. Both require business ownership skills that medical training doesn't provide. You have to handle marketing, patient acquisition, operations, and the reality that a patient leaving your panel is revenue walking out the door. That's a different kind of stress than employed medicine, but it's a stress you control.

If you're a primary care physician seriously considering DPC, the practical starting point is researching the DPC Alliance, which publishes toolkits and practice data. Talk to physicians who have made the transition, not just the advocates but also the ones who found it harder than expected. Model your financial projections conservatively. And don't launch until you have your Runway Number at twelve months or more, because the ramp-up period before a DPC practice reaches full membership capacity typically runs six to eighteen months.

Building Income That Doesn't Depend on One Employer

Financial sovereignty has two levers: reducing your burn rate and building income sources that aren't controlled by a single employer. The second lever is where most physicians haven't looked yet.

Your medical knowledge, your clinical judgment, and your credential are assets. An asset can generate income in more than one way. The system you're working inside has trained you to think of your MD as something that belongs to a practice or hospital. It doesn't. It belongs to you.

Physicians are increasingly building supplemental income streams that don't require a full pivot out of clinical medicine. Medical-legal consulting is one of the more accessible entry points. Attorneys on both plaintiff and defense sides need physician reviewers who can assess cases, write reports, and testify. The work is asynchronous, the hourly rates are strong, and the skills transfer directly from clinical training. A single medical-legal case can generate income equivalent to several clinic sessions with none of the patient care overhead.

Medical writing and clinical content development is another path. Pharmaceutical companies, medical device firms, health technology companies, and continuing medical education organizations all hire physicians to write, review, and validate clinical content. This work is often done on a project basis, doesn't require leaving your current position, and builds a portfolio that can expand over time.

Telemedicine shifts, done through platforms that credential you independently of your main employer, provide a second income stream with scheduling flexibility. Some physicians use weekend telemedicine shifts specifically to accelerate runway fund building without changing their primary position.

These aren't presented as a portfolio career plan. That's Chapter 17's territory. The point here is narrower. Even a single additional income stream that generates $2,000 to $5,000 per month changes your financial position meaningfully. It shortens the time to reach your target Runway Number. It reduces the psychological weight of dependence on one employer. And it gives you something to expand if the primary position becomes untenable.

The principle is simple: every dollar of income that doesn't come from your main employer is a dollar of leverage your employer doesn't control.

The Financial Freedom Worksheet

The Financial Freedom Worksheet is a tool you build once and update quarterly. It's a single document, not a complicated spreadsheet. It has five components.

Current Runway Number. Your liquid assets divided by your essential monthly expenses. Update this number every quarter. Track whether it's going up or down.

Monthly essential expense floor. The minimum you need to cover true essentials. This is the number your runway calculation uses. Keep it separated from your total burn rate so you can see the gap clearly.

Overhead reduction target. Identify the specific line items you're targeting for reduction. Put dollar amounts and timelines on them. Vague intentions don't move numbers.

Runway fund balance and target. A dedicated savings account earmarked for runway only. Name it something clear in your banking app so you don't accidentally fold it into general savings. Set a target balance that represents twelve months of essential expenses. Track monthly progress toward it.

Supplemental income tracker. List any income sources outside your primary employer. Include the amount, the time investment, and whether it's active or in development. Even if this column is blank right now, the act of looking at it monthly keeps the question alive.

You don't need a financial advisor to build this worksheet. You need honesty and about two hours on a Saturday morning with your bank statements in front of you. Do it once, correctly. Then update it every three months. Physicians who run this quarterly tend to hit their Runway Number target faster than they expected, because the tracking itself changes spending behavior in ways that a vague goal doesn't.

What Sovereignty Actually Changes

When your Runway Number crosses twelve months, something shifts in how you hold your job.

A difficult administrator becomes a problem to solve rather than a threat to your survival. A contract renewal negotiation becomes a conversation you can walk away from if the terms don't work. A toxic colleague or a dysfunctional leadership team becomes a reason to look elsewhere rather than a permanent condition you have no choice but to absorb. A call schedule that's destroying your health becomes something you can push back on rather than silently accept.

The physics of the situation change because your dependence changes. You're still in the same job. The external environment hasn't shifted. But your relationship to it has, because you know you can leave. And the knowledge that you can leave is often what gives you the steadiness to stay on your terms rather than theirs.

This isn't a fantasy. It's a practical consequence of building financial cushion. Physicians who've gone through this describe it as the first time in their careers that they felt like professionals rather than employees. They hadn't changed hospitals. They hadn't cut their hours. They'd just stopped being trapped by the math.

Sovereignty doesn't solve every problem. It doesn't fix a genuinely toxic system, and it doesn't replace the structural reforms that Chapter 15 covers. But it restores the one thing that a burned-out physician most needs: real choices.

Your Next Move

Financial sovereignty doesn't require a perfect plan. It requires a starting calculation and one specific action.

This week, run your Runway Number. Pull your last three bank and credit card statements. Total your liquid assets. Divide. Write the number down. If it's under six, that's your baseline and your target is to double it in the next twelve months. If it's over twelve, you're in a stronger position than you think.

Pick one overhead item to cut or reduce this month. One. Put the savings into a dedicated account and label it your runway fund.

Identify one potential supplemental income category that your clinical training supports. Medical-legal. Medical writing. Telemedicine. Teaching. You don't have to launch anything yet. Just research it enough to know whether it fits your situation. That's the beginning of the second income lever.

Then update your Financial Freedom Worksheet at the end of each quarter. Track the number. Watch it move. The gap between where you are and twelve months of freedom almost always closes faster than physicians expect once the calculation is real and visible.

Your degree belongs to you. So does your financial future. Both are worth protecting with the same rigor you'd bring to a complex clinical case.

Stay, Fight, Modify, or Leave: The Four-Path Triage Model

You've spent the first thirteen chapters of this book building a case. You know what burnout is and what it isn't. You've seen how the system captures physicians through contracts, RVUs, inbox overload, prior authorization, and cultural guilt. You've looked at the financial numbers, the mental health barriers, and the quiet ways the profession has been stripped of its autonomy. You've earned the right to make a decision.

So make one.

Not someday. Not after the next review cycle. Not once you've paid off another chunk of student debt. Now. With what you know right now.

The problem is that most burned-out physicians don't have a framework for deciding. They have feelings. They have exhaustion. They have a vague sense that something has to change, followed immediately by a wave of guilt for even thinking it. They stay stuck in the gap between "I can't keep doing this" and "I don't know what else to do."

The Four-Path Burnout Triage Model exists to close that gap.

It's a decision tool, not a personality quiz. It won't tell you who you are or what you're worth. It will help you sort through your current reality, your financial position, your tolerance for conflict, and your appetite for change, and point you toward the path that fits your actual situation. Four paths. Real options. No judgment about which one you pick.

The Triage Model Explained

Triage comes from emergency medicine. When patients come through the door all at once, you don't treat them in the order they arrived. You assess severity, available resources, and likely outcomes, and you prioritize accordingly. You make a decision under pressure with incomplete information because waiting for perfect information costs lives.

Your career is in the same room right now.

The Four-Path Triage Model works the same way. You assess your current state, your resources, and your options. Then you choose a path and move. The four paths are:

Path One: Stay/Repair. You stay in your current role or a similar clinical role, and you actively work to change the conditions driving your distress. You use the tools in this book, set boundaries, renegotiate, organize, and push back. You believe the environment can shift, and you have enough energy and leverage to push.

Path Two: Stay/Shrink. You stay in clinical medicine but reduce your exposure to the parts that are breaking you. You cut hours, change your panel, shed administrative responsibilities, shift to a lower-volume model, or restructure your schedule. You stop trying to fix the system and start managing your contact with it.

Path Three: Lateral Move. You stay inside medicine but exit your current role. You move to a different employer, a different specialty focus, a different care model, or a non-traditional clinical setting. This could mean locums, direct primary care, concierge, telehealth, urgent care, or a hybrid arrangement. You're changing position, not career.

Path Four: Exit. You leave clinical medicine entirely, or you reduce clinical work to a minimal slice of your income while building something else. This could mean a full pivot into medical affairs, consulting, industry, health tech, medico-legal work, or any of the portfolio careers covered in Chapter 17. Your MD becomes a tool in a new context.

No path is better than the others. Each one is right for a different physician at a different moment. The goal of triage is to match you to the path that fits your reality, not the one that sounds most impressive at a dinner party.

Path One: Stay/Repair

Stay/Repair makes sense when the core problem is fixable and you still have the will and the leverage to fix it. It requires two things to be true at the same time: the system you're in has some capacity to change, and you have enough capacity left to push.

That's a narrower window than most people think.

If your institution has already demonstrated that leadership will absorb physician concerns, produce a wellness task force, and then do nothing, Stay/Repair is probably not the right path for you. You're not failing to push hard enough. The system you're in has decided that physician complaints are a PR problem, not an operations problem. Pushing harder won't change that calculus.

Stay/Repair works when you have genuine institutional leverage. That means you're in a position where your departure would cost the organization enough that they'd rather negotiate than replace you. It means there are other physicians around you willing to stand together. It means you've read Chapter 11 on the power of no and you're ready to use it as a real tool, not a thought experiment.

If those conditions exist, the Stay/Repair path is active and specific. You document your current workload against your contract benchmarks. You identify the three to five specific changes that would materially reduce your distress, and you put them in writing. You request a formal meeting with administration, not an informal chat. You bring data. You make clear what you're asking for and what happens if the request isn't addressed. Then you follow through.

This path also includes organizing with colleagues. If a policy is driving collective harm, one physician raising it is a complaint. Five physicians raising it with documented evidence is a governance issue. Chapter 15 covers this in depth. The point here is that Stay/Repair is a collective action path as much as an individual negotiation path. Solo physicians rarely repair systems. Groups do.

The honest warning: Stay/Repair has a time limit. If you've been pushing for more than twelve months without measurable change, the path isn't working. That doesn't mean you failed. It means the institution has chosen not to change, and you now have better information for your next decision.

Path Two: Stay/Shrink

Stay/Shrink is the most underused path in medicine. Physicians are conditioned to equate reducing their clinical footprint with failure. Cutting hours feels like giving up. Shrinking a panel feels like abandoning patients. Dropping a committee feels like letting colleagues down.

None of that is true.

Shrinking is a resource management decision. You're a physician with a finite amount of capacity. When you're running at 110% for years, you don't produce 110% of the output. You produce degraded work, make more errors, lose clinical sharpness, and eventually burn out completely. Shrinking on purpose before you collapse is smarter clinical management than waiting for the system to break you down to zero.

The Stay/Shrink path is right for you if clinical medicine still holds meaning but the volume, pace, or administrative burden is what's killing you. It's the right path if your financial situation gives you room to reduce income in exchange for reduced load. It's the right path if you've run the Runway Number from Chapter 13 and know you can absorb a schedule reduction without losing your financial floor.

What does Stay/Shrink actually look like?

It looks like dropping from full-time to 0.8 FTE and protecting that 20% as non-negotiable time for your life. It looks like converting to a direct primary care model with a capped panel where you see fewer patients per day and bill them directly instead of drowning in prior authorizations. It looks like transitioning to a concierge model where your income comes from membership fees rather than RVU volume. It looks like accepting a hospitalist schedule that gives you defined blocks off instead of an outpatient schedule that bleeds into every evening.

It also looks like deliberately shedding the add-ons that crept onto your plate without your consent. The quality metrics committee. The wellness ambassador role your employer assigned you as if asking a drowning person to save others. The weekend coverage you said yes to three years ago and never renegotiated. These things aren't required by your medical license. Many of them aren't even required by your contract if you read it carefully with the red-flag checklist from Chapter 9.

Shrinking requires saying no to volume, and institutions will push back. They'll tell you about patient need. They'll tell you there's no one else to fill the gaps. They'll invoke the calling. You've seen all of that language before. The appropriate response is to hold your boundary and to document, in writing, that you made this request and that it was acknowledged.

The financial calculation matters here. A 20% reduction in clinical hours does not have to mean a 20% reduction in total income. If you layer in even one non-clinical income stream, like consulting, expert witness work, a medical education contract, or a small digital product serving physicians, you can offset part of the reduction. Chapter 17 goes deeper on this. The point is that Stay/Shrink is not automatically a financial sacrifice. It depends on how you structure the transition.

Path Three: Lateral Move

Sometimes the problem isn't medicine. Sometimes it's your employer, your specialty, your call structure, or the specific corporate entity that owns your group. A lateral move means you leave your current role but you stay inside clinical practice.

This is the most practically accessible path for physicians who are miserable at their current job but haven't lost their relationship with patient care. The research on physician attrition consistently shows that many physicians who leave one employer would have stayed in medicine if they'd had better options visible to them. They weren't done with medicine. They were done with that specific version of it.

A lateral move might mean:

Going from a hospital-employed outpatient position to a locum tenens arrangement that lets you work on your own terms for two to three years while you figure out what comes next. Locums gets a bad reputation in some circles, but for physicians who need geographic flexibility, schedule control, and a break from the permanent-employment trap, it can be genuinely restorative.

Moving from a PE-owned practice where your autonomy has been systematically stripped to an independent group where physicians still make clinical decisions. These groups are harder to find, but they exist in almost every specialty. You may take a short-term income hit. Many physicians report that the trade is worth it.

Shifting within your specialty to a different care setting. An emergency physician exhausted by the volume and acuity of a Level I trauma center might find that an urgent care setting, a freestanding ED, or a rural critical access hospital changes the experience entirely. A hospitalist burned out on 24-hour shifts might move to a short-stay observation unit or a transitional care role. A primary care physician drowning in a 25-patient-per-day panel might move into a geriatrics practice or a chronic disease management program that allows longer, slower visits.

Starting a direct primary care or concierge practice. This is technically a lateral move into a different care model rather than a different employer. The shift is substantial: you cap your panel, charge directly, eliminate most third-party billing, and reclaim control of your time and clinical decisions. The startup work is real. The financial transition period is real. But the physicians who make this move report high rates of satisfaction precisely because they've taken back the piece of clinical practice that made them want to become physicians in the first place.

The lateral move path requires a clear-eyed look at what you're actually escaping. If the problem is structural to medicine in general, a lateral move won't fix it. If the problem is specific to your employer, your region's market, or a particular practice model, a lateral move might be exactly the right tool. The diagnostic question is: would the same role at a different organization feel different? If the answer is yes, you have a lateral move case.

Path Four: Exit

Exit is the most charged word in this chapter. It carries weight that the other paths don't. Physicians are taught that leaving clinical medicine is a failure of commitment, a betrayal of the profession, and a waste of years of training. None of that framing is accurate, and all of it serves the people who benefit from keeping physicians tethered to jobs that are breaking them.

Exit doesn't mean your training was wasted. It means your training equipped you with a credential and a skill set that has value in multiple contexts, and you're choosing to use it in a context that doesn't require you to work yourself into the ground.

Exit is the right path when clinical medicine has become consistently incompatible with your health, your values, or your life. When every boundary you've set gets overridden. When the moral injury of delivering inadequate care inside a broken system has accumulated past the point where you can separate yourself from it. When the financial math of your current situation makes change more possible than continuing. When you've tried Stay/Repair and Stay/Shrink and you're still not okay.

It's also the right path when something else is pulling you forward with genuine force. A physician who is genuinely excited about medical affairs, health technology, medico-legal consulting, or building a platform for other physicians isn't running away from medicine. They're running toward a new use of the same skills.

The non-clinical sectors actively recruiting physicians in 2026 are substantial. Pharmaceutical and biotech companies need physicians for medical science liaison roles, clinical development, regulatory affairs, and medical affairs leadership. Health technology companies need physician advisors, clinical informaticists, and product leaders who can bridge the gap between engineering and clinical reality. Payer organizations need physician reviewers, utilization management directors, and population health strategists. Management consulting firms need healthcare specialists. Law firms and independent firms need expert witnesses. The medico-legal market for reviewing records, consulting on standards of care, and testifying is active and well-compensated. Chapter 17 covers the full menu.

The exit path doesn't have to be abrupt. Most physicians who successfully transition out of clinical medicine do it in stages. They keep some clinical hours, even a single day per week, while they build the non-clinical income base. They don't resign on a Tuesday and figure out the rest later. They run the 12-Month Transition Calendar from Chapter 18, which maps the practical steps of updating credentials, building a corporate resume, networking into target sectors, and timing the financial shift so they're never crossing a gap without a bridge.

The hardest part of the exit path isn't logistical. It's psychological. Chapter 16 goes deep on decoupling identity from the MD. For now, understand this: choosing exit doesn't mean your years of training were a mistake. It means you're a physician who's now choosing how to deploy that credential on your own terms. That's agency. That's exactly what this book has been building toward.

Running Your Own Triage

Here's how to actually use this model. You don't pick a path by reading the descriptions and feeling a vague resonance with one of them. You run a structured diagnostic.

Work through these four assessment areas:

Your Burnout Severity

Pull out the Burnout Vital Signs checklist from the appendix if you haven't already. Score yourself honestly. Mild to moderate burnout, where you're exhausted but still functional and still find some meaning in your clinical work, is compatible with Stay/Repair or Stay/Shrink. Severe burnout, where you're past caring, making errors you wouldn't have made two years ago, and can't remember the last time a clinical interaction felt rewarding, is a signal that the higher-intensity paths, Lateral Move or Exit, deserve real weight. You can't repair a system from a position of complete depletion.

Your Financial Position

You calculated your Runway Number in Chapter 13. Use it here. If your Runway Number is less than six months, your options are constrained by real financial risk. You may need to prioritize Stay/Shrink as a bridge while you build reserves, before making a move that involves any income disruption. If your Runway Number is twelve months or more, you have genuine optionality. You can afford to take the time to run a careful lateral move or exit transition without panic-selling your next career move.

Your Institutional Reality

Look at your current environment without the benefit of the doubt. Has leadership demonstrated any capacity to change in response to physician feedback in the past two years? If yes, and if you have leverage, Stay/Repair is worth a defined, time-limited attempt. If the answer is no, or if you work for a PE-owned entity where the financial model depends on physician volume and there's no structural incentive to reduce it, Stay/Repair is a very long bet. Be honest here. Wishful thinking about institutional change is how physicians lose another three years.

Your Clinical Relationship

Do you still want to practice medicine? Somewhere underneath the exhaustion, the inbox, and the prior authorizations, is there a version of clinical practice you'd want to do if the conditions were right? If yes, that's information. It points toward Stay paths or Lateral Move. If the honest answer is no, that you're genuinely done with patient care and you're staying only because you don't see an alternative, that's also information. It points toward Exit, and it's not a character flaw. It's a signal that the system has finally extracted more than it gave back.

Once you've answered those four questions, the path with the most evidence behind it becomes clearer. You might find that two paths are close, say Stay/Shrink and Lateral Move. That's fine. Pick one, run it for six months, and assess. The model isn't a one-time decision tool. It's a framework you can return to as your circumstances change.

Writing It Down

The triage process only works if you're honest with yourself, and honesty on this topic is easier when it's on paper. Write out your answers to the four assessment areas. Write out which path you're choosing and why. Write down the three specific actions you'll take in the next thirty days to move that path forward.

That last part matters. The path you choose has to produce action within thirty days. Choosing a path and then continuing to operate exactly as before isn't triage. It's the same avoidance pattern dressed in new language.

For Stay/Repair: your thirty-day action is to identify the specific change you're requesting and put it in writing to administration, with a follow-up meeting scheduled.

For Stay/Shrink: your thirty-day action is to calculate the income math on a schedule reduction, identify what you'd drop first, and make a request or take a step toward a different practice model.

For Lateral Move: your thirty-day action is to identify three specific roles or settings you'd consider and reach out to at least one person who works in one of them.

For Exit: your thirty-day action is to identify one non-clinical sector that interests you, research the typical physician entry points, and have a single conversation with a physician who's already made the move.

None of these actions commit you to anything permanent. They commit you to gathering real information instead of staying paralyzed.

What If You Change Your Mind?

You're allowed to. Triage isn't a tattoo. If you start down Stay/Repair and realize after six months that the institution isn't budging, you move to Lateral Move. If you begin a concierge transition and find that it's not solving the underlying problem, you revisit your assessment. The model is built for iteration because careers are dynamic and the healthcare system keeps changing around you.

The goal isn't to make the perfect decision on the first try. The goal is to stop drifting in the current and start swimming in a direction you've actually chosen.

Physicians are trained to tolerate a lot. Long hours, delayed gratification, hierarchical pressure, patient suffering, system failure. That training is real and it's been useful. But it's also made many physicians extraordinarily good at absorbing conditions that would cause anyone else to change course immediately. You've been tolerating the intolerable and calling it professionalism.

You now have four paths and a diagnostic tool. The question on the table isn't whether things are bad enough to warrant a change. You already answered that. The question is which change makes sense given your current reality.

Pick a path. Write it down. Take one action in thirty days.

That's triage.

Your Next Move

Three things to do before you finish this chapter:

1. Score yourself on the four assessment areas (burnout severity, financial position, institutional reality, clinical relationship) and write the answers down. Use actual words, not mental notes. Mental notes evaporate.

1. Identify which path has the most evidence behind it. If two are close, pick the one that involves the first action you can actually take in the next two weeks.

1. Name your thirty-day action for the path you've chosen and put it in your calendar as an appointment with a specific deliverable. A scheduled action with a deliverable is different from an intention. Intentions don't move careers. Scheduled deliverables do.

The next two chapters build on what you've decided here. Chapter 15 covers collective action for physicians who are choosing Stay paths and want structural leverage. Chapter 16 addresses the identity work that makes every path, including the ones that feel like staying, genuinely sustainable for the long term.

Collective Action: The Profession Remembers Its Power

Every strategy in this book up to now has been about what you can do alone. You can audit your contract, calculate your Runway Number, set boundaries, seek safe mental health support, and run your own four-path triage. Those moves matter. They protect you. But there's a ceiling on what any single physician can accomplish by working solo against a system designed by lawyers, administrators, and shareholders who have been coordinating for decades.

This chapter is about something they don't want you to think about: your collective power.

Physicians are among the most educated, most credentialed workers in the country. They are also among the least organized. That's not an accident. Corporate health systems have actively benefited from keeping doctors isolated, competing, and too exhausted to compare notes with the colleague across the hall. The culture of medicine reinforces it. You were trained to solve problems individually. Speaking up felt like complaining. Organizing felt like politics. And politics, you were told, had no place in medicine.

That framing served the people at the top of the org chart. It didn't serve you.

The profession hasn't forgotten its power. It's just been too tired to use it. This chapter is about how to start using it again, strategically and without blowing up your career in the process.

Staff Bylaws and Institutional Rights

Most physicians have never read their medical staff bylaws.

That's understandable. They're long, dense, and written in a language that reads like a legal contract designed to discourage you from finishing it. But inside those bylaws are rights that already belong to you, rights that hospitals and health systems would rather you never invoke.

Medical staff bylaws govern the relationship between the physician workforce and the hospital or health system. They typically spell out how departments are structured, how medical staff meetings work, how peer review is conducted, how department chiefs are selected, and under what conditions the medical staff can call for a review of administrative decisions. In many institutions, those bylaws also give the medical staff the right to vote on certain operational changes, to formally appeal credentialing decisions, and to elect their own leadership.

Here's what matters: in most hospitals, the medical staff is technically a separate legal entity from the hospital administration. The medical staff elects its own officers. It has its own bylaws. It has standing to raise formal concerns through channels that are harder for administration to simply ignore or dismiss.

Most physicians don't use any of this.

When a hospital cuts call pay, adds unfunded administrative duties, or quietly changes RVU thresholds, the typical physician response is private frustration. Maybe a venting session in the break room. Maybe a scathing anonymous comment on a survey that no one reads. The system counts on that.

Using your medical staff bylaws changes the dynamic. It forces formal process. It creates a paper trail. It puts administration in the position of having to respond in writing to concerns raised through legitimate channels, rather than brushing off hallway complaints.

Start by getting a copy of your institution's medical staff bylaws. They are typically available through the medical staff office. If they're not easily accessible, that itself is worth noting. Read the sections on medical staff meetings, member rights, and any provisions about administrative accountability. Find out when meetings happen and whether physicians outside of department leadership can bring items to the floor.

Then find out who your elected medical staff officers are and whether they actually represent the interests of working physicians or have become administrators by another name. Many chief medical officers started in elected medical staff positions and then got absorbed into administration. They wear two hats and serve one master. Knowing who in your medical staff leadership is genuinely independent matters.

The goal isn't to file grievances for sport. The goal is to stop pretending that informal channels are your only option when they clearly aren't working.

Medical Unions: What They Are and What They Can Do

The word "union" still makes some physicians flinch. It carries baggage. It sounds like something for factory workers, not physicians. It feels at odds with the professional identity most of you spent a decade building.

Set that aside for a moment and look at what's actually happened.

Hospital systems have consolidated. Private equity owns physician groups across specialties. Administrators outnumber doctors by ratios that would have been unthinkable thirty years ago. Pay compression is real. Workload creep is real. The power imbalance between a physician employed by a large health system and the health system itself is enormous. Physicians negotiating individually against a corporate entity with a legal team and an HR department built specifically for these situations are at a structural disadvantage.

Unions exist to correct that imbalance.

In some states and some specialties, physician unionization is already underway. Resident physicians have been organizing for years through organizations like the Committee of Interns and Residents, which is affiliated with the Service Employees International Union. Attending physicians in some academic medical centers and public hospital systems have also organized successfully. The legal framework for physician unionization depends heavily on employment status and state law, but the pathway exists and has been used.

What can collective bargaining actually accomplish for physicians? The honest answer is: it depends on what physicians are willing to organize around and how well they can maintain solidarity through the negotiation process. But in settings where it's worked, collective bargaining has produced enforceable limits on call burdens, mandatory processes before workload changes can be implemented, transparency requirements around compensation models, and protections against retaliation for physicians who raise patient safety concerns.

Those aren't small wins. They're the kinds of protections that prevent the contract creep and workload expansion covered in Chapter 9 from happening silently and without recourse.

There are real limitations too. If you're classified as a management employee, or if you work in certain private practice structures, traditional labor law may not cover you the same way it covers employed hospital physicians. The rules differ by state. Retaliation, while illegal, happens. Organizing takes time and energy that burned-out physicians often don't have in reserve.

But the option deserves a serious look, not a reflexive dismissal. If you're employed by a large health system and you've watched your working conditions deteriorate year over year with no mechanism for pushback, collective bargaining is worth researching as a structural tool, not a radical act.

The first concrete step is to find out your employment classification. Are you employed directly by the hospital? A physician management company? A private equity-backed group? Your classification affects what organizing options are available to you. Talk to an employment attorney who works with physicians before making any moves at work. Know the legal landscape before you speak up internally.

Voting Blocs and Professional Organizations

Unions aren't the only mechanism for collective physician power. Professional organizations have existed for over a century, and while many physicians have written them off as bureaucratic institutions that produce position statements no one reads, some of them still carry real leverage when physicians actually show up and use them.

The American Medical Association is the most visible national organization, but it's also the most diluted in terms of any single physician's influence. State medical associations and specialty societies are often where physician organizing has more traction and more direct impact on the policy decisions that affect day-to-day practice.

State medical associations lobby legislatures on scope of practice laws, prior authorization reform, noncompete enforcement, and Medicaid reimbursement. They file amicus briefs. They support or oppose legislation that directly affects whether physicians can practice with some measure of autonomy or whether every clinical decision gets filtered through a corporate approval chain. When physicians don't show up, don't vote in organizational elections, and don't engage with the policy process, that space gets filled by hospital lobbyists and insurance industry representatives who have been working those relationships full-time for years.

The prior authorization data cited earlier in this book (Chapter 2) exists partly because organized medicine has pushed for data collection and reporting. The legislative efforts to reduce prior authorization burdens in multiple states happened because physician organizations built coalitions, showed up at committee hearings, and put sustained pressure on legislators over multiple sessions. That's collective action working through existing channels, and it produces real results even when the pace is frustrating.

Within specialty societies, the same dynamic applies at a smaller, faster-moving scale. If your specialty organization is discussing practice guidelines that will affect your workload, your clinical autonomy, or your ability to bill for services, your vote in that organization's leadership elections matters. Your presence at the annual meeting's business sessions matters. Your willingness to serve on a committee matters. Most specialty society committees have vacancies because most physicians are too busy to fill them.

Here's the part that gets overlooked: specialty societies often have direct relationships with payers and accreditation bodies. When a specialty society pushes back formally on an insurer's coverage policy or on a prior authorization requirement, it carries more institutional weight than an individual physician complaint. Organized specialty voices have gotten coverage policies revised. They've gotten prior authorization requirements modified for specific procedures. They've influenced CMS rulemaking in ways that individual physicians never could.

This doesn't mean throwing yourself into committee work as an escape from your own career decisions. Chapter 14 gave you a framework for deciding your personal path. This chapter is about recognizing that your individual path and the profession's collective health are connected. Physicians who stay and fight need the system to change, not just their own corner of it. Physicians who modify their roles still work within an infrastructure that's shaped by policy. Even physicians who exit into non-clinical careers often return to consulting or advisory roles where the state of medicine matters.

Joining and actively participating in your state medical association and your specialty society costs time, but it's time that puts you in the room where decisions affecting your profession are made. That's a different kind of leverage than anything you can accomplish alone.

Building Solidarity Without Burning Bridges

Collective action requires trust. And trust requires conversations that most physicians have been trained to avoid.

Talking to colleagues about working conditions feels risky. Medicine's culture of individual stoicism (the same culture that makes physicians reluctant to seek mental health support, as discussed in Chapter 12) also makes physicians reluctant to say out loud that the system isn't working. Complaining, comparing notes, asking what the doctor down the hall is being paid. These feel like violations of a professional code. They're not. They're the basic information-sharing that every other organized workforce considers standard.

Salary transparency is especially important. Physician pay within the same institution, the same department, and sometimes the same job description varies in ways that many physicians have no idea about. Corporate employers benefit from this opacity. When you don't know what your colleagues earn, you can't negotiate from a realistic baseline. You also can't recognize when you're being paid below market specifically because the system knows you won't ask.

Talking to colleagues doesn't require a formal meeting or a dramatic disclosure. It can start with simple questions. "Did your workload change when they rolled out the new panel expansion?" "How are you handling the prior auth burden for [specialty-specific procedure]?" "Did you negotiate your last contract or did you just sign it?" These conversations build a shared picture of what's actually happening. They break the isolation that keeps each physician thinking their problems are personal rather than systemic.

The risk of retaliation for these conversations is real and varies significantly by institution. Some systems are more tolerant of physician organizing than others. Some department chiefs actively suppress it. If you're in a culture where you know retaliation is likely, be thoughtful about who you talk to and in what context. Start with colleagues you already trust. Keep conversations private until there's enough critical mass to have safety in numbers.

When it comes to formal collective action inside an institution, there are specific ways to reduce personal exposure. Raising concerns through the medical staff bylaws process is less personally exposed than sending an individual complaint email, because it uses institutional channels rather than creating an individual record of dissent. Submitting concerns through formal patient safety reporting mechanisms has legal protections in many states that individual complaints don't. Organizing a group of physicians to jointly request a meeting with administration is harder to ignore and harder to retaliate against than one physician asking alone.

You don't have to be the loudest voice in the room to contribute to collective action. Showing up to a medical staff meeting when there's an important vote counts. Voting in your specialty society elections counts. Signing onto a letter from your state medical association counts. Talking to one colleague about their contract experience counts. These aren't heroic gestures. They're small acts of coordination that add up.

The physicians who have pushed back successfully against predatory practice conditions, who have won transparency, negotiated protections, or changed institutional policy, rarely did it by being uniquely brave individuals. They did it because they found colleagues who shared their concerns and were willing to act together. That's how collective power actually works.

What Institutional Leverage Actually Looks Like

Leverage inside an institution comes from a few specific places: your scarcity value, your patient relationships, your referral patterns, and your medical staff standing.

Physician scarcity is a real factor in many specialties and many markets. If your specialty is in short supply in your region, your employer knows that replacing you is expensive and time-consuming. That's leverage you rarely use because no one teaches you to think about it that way. Knowing your market value (something Chapter 13 touched on in the context of financial sovereignty) isn't just about negotiating your own compensation. It's about understanding what your departure or collective departure by a group of physicians would actually cost the system.

Patient relationships are leverage too. Patients follow physicians. When physicians leave a practice, a significant percentage of their established patients follow them or choose to find care elsewhere rather than seeing whoever fills the position. Hospital systems and large groups know this. It affects how seriously they take physician concerns, particularly among high-volume clinicians with established panels.

Referral patterns matter in markets where physicians retain some ability to direct where their patients go for specialty or ancillary services. When a health system's practices generate friction, physicians route referrals elsewhere if they have options. Administrators notice this in the revenue data even when they don't explicitly acknowledge the connection.

Medical staff standing and the formal rights it creates have already been covered in the bylaws section above. But it's worth connecting these dots: institutional leverage is strongest when physicians use multiple mechanisms together. The department that raises formal concerns through the bylaws process, while key members consult employment attorneys, while the group signals clearly that working conditions affect their ability to maintain their patient panels, is a department that administration has to take seriously. That's not a single angry physician who can be managed, reassured, or waited out. It's a coordinated response.

None of this requires a confrontational posture. The most effective collective action inside institutions tends to be matter-of-fact: here is the problem, here is what it's costing in physician retention and patient access, here is what needs to change, here is the timeline we expect. That's a business conversation, delivered by people who understand the system they're operating in. Administrators respond to business cases more reliably than they respond to moral arguments.

Your Next Move

Pick one. Don't try to tackle all of this at once.

If you've never read your medical staff bylaws, that's your first action. Get them, read the sections on member rights and medical staff meetings, and put the next meeting date on your calendar.

If you've been operating without knowing what your colleagues earn or how their working conditions compare to yours, start one conversation this week. Pick someone you trust. Ask a genuine question about their experience with something specific: call burden, inbox volume, contract terms. Just start.

If you're not a member of your state medical association or your primary specialty society, join. Then actually look at the leadership structure. Find out when elections happen and who's running. Even showing up to vote is a more active role than most physician members play.

If collective action inside your institution feels relevant to your situation, consult an employment attorney before taking any formal steps. Know your legal protections. Understand your employment classification. Don't organize blind.

The system that's breaking physicians didn't get this powerful overnight. It got here because the people running it coordinated while physicians worked in isolation. Reversing that takes time, and it starts with small acts of connection. Find the colleagues who see what you see. Compare notes. Show up. The profession has more power than it's been using. It just needs physicians willing to remember that.

Decoupling Identity from the MD

The first time someone asks what you do and your mouth goes dry before answering, you understand something most physicians never put into words. The question is about work. The feeling underneath it is about worth.

For most doctors, the MD credential isn't just a professional title. It's the organizing principle of everything. It's the reason you didn't sleep in your twenties. It's the frame that held your sacrifice together. It's the answer to the question of who you are when everything else feels uncertain. When that credential gets connected to a system that's grinding you down, you end up in an impossible position: staying destroys you, but leaving feels like erasing yourself.

That's the grip you need to loosen before anything else in Part IV can work.

Decoupling your identity from the MD doesn't mean abandoning medicine, rejecting the work you did, or pretending the training didn't matter. It means building a sense of self that can survive any employment decision you make. It means being a physician without being owned by the credential. It means having an answer to "who are you?" that doesn't collapse the moment your clinical role changes.

The Sunk-Cost Fallacy in Medical Identity

You know what a sunk cost is. You teach it, in a way, every time you talk to a patient who stayed in a bad situation too long because of how much they'd already invested. The costs already paid can't be recovered. The only rational question is what happens next.

Knowing that doesn't make it easy when the sunk costs belong to you.

Physicians have sunk more into their profession than almost anyone in any field. The math alone is staggering. Four years of undergraduate work, four years of medical school, three to seven years of residency, sometimes additional fellowship years on top of that. In 2026, the average medical student graduates with somewhere between $200,000 and $300,000 in debt. Add the opportunity cost of the income you didn't earn during training years. Add the relationships that frayed under the pressure. Add the health you traded for call nights. Add the personal milestones you postponed because medicine came first.

That's not a small investment. That's a life-defining sacrifice, and the human mind doesn't let go of life-defining sacrifices easily.

When the system that's supposed to honor that sacrifice instead treats you as a billing unit, something locks up. The cognitive dissonance is intense. If you can acknowledge that the system is broken and still stay without fighting for change, it means the sacrifice was possibly in service of something that doesn't deserve it. If you consider leaving, it means the sacrifice might not have bought what you thought it would. Either conclusion is uncomfortable. So many physicians do neither: they stay, they suffer, and they tell themselves the suffering is the price of the work.

It isn't. The suffering is the price of not separating who you are from what you do.

The sunk-cost fallacy in medical identity sounds like this: "I spent too much to walk away now." It sounds like: "If I stop practicing, what was the point of all that training?" It sounds like: "Medicine is the only thing I'm good at." And under all of those thoughts is the same assumption: that the value of your past investment is measured by how long you continue in the same direction, regardless of what that direction costs you now.

That assumption is wrong. The value of your training isn't destroyed by a career change or a role modification. Your clinical knowledge doesn't evaporate. Your diagnostic thinking doesn't disappear. Your ability to communicate risk, read research, and understand human suffering doesn't stop existing because you're no longer seeing

28 patients a day. Those capacities travel with you. They belong to you, not to your employer.

The question isn't whether you've paid enough to justify staying. The question is what you're actually buying with the years you still have left.

Who You Are Without the White Coat

Most physicians have never seriously asked this question. Not because they're shallow, but because medicine crowds everything else out. The training culture demands total immersion. You're expected to make medicine your world, and if you do that long enough, you can lose track of what else exists.

So try this: write down five things that are true about you that have nothing to do with medicine. Not "I'm hardworking" (that came from medicine). Not "I'm good under pressure" (that came from medicine too). Things that existed before your first day of med school, or that developed in the margins that training left open.

Most physicians struggle with this. A few manage it. The ones who can name five non-clinical truths about themselves tend to be the ones who navigate career transitions without falling apart.

If you can't do it easily, that's information. It tells you how much of your identity construction happened inside a single institution, a single role, a single credential. It also tells you where the reconstruction work needs to happen.

Here's where to look.

Your values don't live inside clinical medicine. They live inside you and get expressed through clinical medicine, but they'd find expression elsewhere too. If you're driven by justice, that doesn't go away when you stop seeing patients. If you're energized by solving hard problems, that skill set exists in a dozen non-clinical settings. If you care about people in a way that runs bone-deep, a credential change doesn't switch that off. Values are durable. Roles are not.

Your skills extend much further than you think. Physicians are trained to gather incomplete information quickly, form a hypothesis, test it, and revise the plan when new evidence appears. That's not a medical skill. That's a thinking skill that most industries would pay well for. You can read a research paper and know whether the methodology is sound. You can explain a complicated risk to someone who's scared and confused. You can manage situations where the stakes are high and the information is imperfect. These are rare capabilities. The medical system has convinced you they're only valuable inside a clinical setting. They're not.

Your relationships don't require your role to stay intact. The people who care about you do so because of who you are, not because you have a stethoscope. This sounds obvious. But physicians who have built most of their social world inside medicine sometimes discover that their identity and their social network are tied together in ways that make any change feel like a double loss. Separating those threads is worth doing before any major transition.

Your curiosity predates your degree. Whatever drew you to medicine in the first place, whether it was the science, the human contact, the problem-solving, or the desire to do something that mattered, that curiosity existed before you were accepted to medical school. It can exist after whatever comes next too.

None of this erases what the white coat meant. It meant a great deal. It still does. The goal here is to stop letting it mean everything, because when it means everything, the system that employs you holds total power over your sense of self. And as you've seen across the previous fifteen chapters, that system will use that power without hesitation.

Grief as Part of the Process

This part doesn't get talked about enough. When physicians modify their clinical role significantly, or exit clinical medicine altogether, many experience something that feels like loss. That's because it is loss.

You're not losing who you are. You are losing a particular version of yourself that you spent years building, a version that operated inside a specific set of rituals, relationships, and routines that had their own meaning. The smell of a hospital, the rhythm of morning rounds, the particular weight of a patient trusting you with something they've never told anyone else, those experiences carry real significance. Walking away from them, even voluntarily, even when staying was slowly destroying you, involves a real reckoning.

Some physicians feel this as relief with an undercurrent of guilt. Some feel it as grief that surprises them with its sharpness. Some cycle between the two. All of it is normal. All of it is a sign that what you did mattered, and that you're paying honest attention to the change you're making.

What tends to make this worse is when the grief gets suppressed or treated as weakness. The same culture that told you asking for help was a liability also tends to treat grief over career change as self-indulgence. You're supposed to pivot smartly and move forward efficiently. Feeling sad about it means you didn't fully commit to the new direction.

That framing is unhelpful. Grief doesn't indicate ambivalence. Grieving what you're leaving is actually how you leave it cleanly. Physicians who skip this step often find it waiting for them later, usually at an inconvenient time, usually dressed up as something else.

What does healthy processing look like here? Not performative suffering, not obsessive rumination. More like intentional acknowledgment. You can name what you're losing specifically. The continuity of long-term patient relationships. The identity shorthand that a medical title provides in any room. The sense of doing something that most people around you can't do. The particular satisfaction of making a correct diagnosis. The camaraderie of a good team. Name these things clearly. They're real losses. Honoring them doesn't mean you made the wrong choice.

There's also something worth naming at the other end. When physicians get enough distance from a role that was breaking them, many describe a version of something they didn't expect. The relief doesn't just feel like exhaustion lifting. It feels like remembering who they were before the system got its hands on them. That's not a small thing to look forward to.

One more piece: grief has a timeline, but the timeline is individual. Some physicians feel settled in a new direction within six months. Others take two or three years to fully integrate the change. If you're in a transition and it's taking longer than you expected, that doesn't mean something is wrong. It means you're doing something significant, and significant changes take time to land.

Building a Values-Based Identity Architecture

Once you understand that the white coat isn't the load-bearing wall of your personality, you can start building something more durable. The goal is a sense of self that's grounded in what you value, what you're capable of, and how you want to spend your time, rather than in a title, an employer, or a set of procedures.

This isn't about self-help exercises. It's practical construction. Here's how to do it.

Start with the values inventory. Get specific. "Helping people" is too vague to build anything on. What kind of helping? At what scale? In what form? If you value precision, that shows up differently than if you value connection. If you value teaching, that's a different path than if you value creating. Push past the first answer to the second and third. The deeper you go, the more usable the output becomes.

Ask yourself which parts of clinical medicine you would miss and which parts you'd never think about again. The parts you'd miss point directly at values. The parts you'd never think about again tell you what you've been doing out of obligation rather than alignment. Both lists are important.

Identify your transferable skills in plain language. Write these down as a working professional would describe them, not the way a CV does. A CV says "managed a panel of 1,800 patients." In transferable language, that's: managed high-stakes relationships with hundreds of people simultaneously, with responsibility for outcomes and accountability for quality. A CV says "performed 400 surgical procedures." In transferable language: developed and executed complex technical processes with near-zero tolerance for error, in high-pressure environments, with incomplete information.

This reframing matters because your brain is still sorting your experience as "medical experience." The rest of the world sorts it as human experience. The translation isn't dumbing it down. It's making it legible to people who can open doors you didn't know existed.

Choose anchoring activities that reinforce a broader identity. If your whole schedule is clinical work, your whole identity becomes clinical. Physicians who successfully maintain a broader sense of self usually have at least one or two regular activities outside of medicine that demand something real from them. A project. A creative pursuit. An intellectual interest. A physical practice. A community involvement. The specific activity matters less than the fact that it's separate from medicine and that it's genuine.

These activities serve a purpose beyond enjoyment. They become evidence, visible to you, that you exist and contribute and belong in spaces that have nothing to do with your clinical role. That evidence accumulates. Over time, it changes how you answer the question "who are you?" even before any formal transition happens.

Rebuild the narrative around your degree. The framing that's been doing damage is this: "I am a doctor." The framing that creates more room is this: "I have a medical degree and a set of skills I can deploy in multiple directions." The first version collapses your identity into a role. The second version positions you as a capable person with portable assets.

This isn't a semantic trick. Language shapes how we think about possibility. Physicians who have internalized "I am a doctor" as their core identity often describe a visceral resistance to considering non-clinical work, not because the work doesn't interest them, but because it feels like a category error. "I'm a doctor. Doctors do clinical work." The second framing loosens that lock. "I have a medical degree. What's the best use of it right now?"

Build relationships outside your clinical world deliberately. When your entire professional network is inside medicine, your sense of what's possible gets limited by what the people around you have done. Talking to physicians who've made lateral moves or full exits, to people in the fields you're curious about, to entrepreneurs, consultants, and executives who work with medical knowledge in non-clinical ways, changes the landscape of what feels real and achievable. It also starts building the network that Chapter 18 will depend on.

You don't need to announce anything. You can explore casually. The exploration itself is part of building a wider identity.

Give yourself permission to be in process. Physicians are trained to reach diagnoses. Uncertainty is a phase you move through to get to an answer. Career identity work doesn't operate on the same timeline. You might spend six months genuinely unsure of what you want next, and that uncertainty is not a failure of decision-making. It's what reconstruction looks like from the inside.

The pressure to have a clear answer, to know your next move, to explain yourself to colleagues and family, is real. But making a premature choice to escape the discomfort of uncertainty often leads to landing in a new role that doesn't fit any better than the one you left. Better to sit with the uncertainty a little longer, with intention, than to sprint toward a decision that resets the clock on a broken situation.

Your Next Move

Before moving to Chapter 17 and the practical shape of a portfolio career, spend time with these four actions. They're not dramatic. But they're the foundation that makes everything else in Part IV stable.

1. Write the two lists. What would you miss from clinical medicine? What would you never think about again? Be honest and specific. Twenty items on each list if you can manage it. The patterns that emerge from those lists are more informative than any assessment tool you could take.

1. Translate three clinical experiences into transferable language. Pick three things you've done in clinical medicine that you're genuinely proud of. Rewrite each one as a capabilities statement that a non-physician hiring manager or collaborator could immediately understand and value. This exercise alone tends to shift how physicians see their own professional worth.

1. Identify two anchoring activities outside medicine and schedule them. Not aspirationally. On the calendar, with a recurring date. They don't have to be elaborate. They have to be real and they have to happen.

1. Have one conversation with someone who has made a move you're curious about. A former colleague who left clinical medicine. A physician who moved into consulting or pharma or a startup. A doctor who went part-time and built something else alongside their clinical work. One real conversation changes the abstract into the possible in a way that no amount of research replicates.

Your degree is real. The training was real. The sacrifice was real. None of that stops being true the moment you stop organizing your entire identity around the credential.

You can carry the knowledge, the skills, and the clinical judgment into whatever comes next. You just don't have to let the system that employed those skills also own your sense of self.

That's the deal worth renegotiating. And you have more leverage than you think.

The 2026 Portfolio Career

The word "portfolio" used to belong to investors and artists. Investors spread money across different assets so no single bad bet could wipe them out. Artists kept a portfolio because their work didn't fit one box. Both groups understood something most physicians were never taught: putting everything into one basket is a risk strategy, not a career strategy.

You went all in on clinical medicine. Your training demanded it. Your identity fused to it, as we covered in Chapter 16. And for a long time, the deal felt fair enough. You gave the system your best years, your sleep, your weekends, and your full attention. In return, you got a salary, a title, and a sense of purpose.

The deal has changed. The system took your best years and kept renegotiating the contract on its own terms. And now a growing number of physicians are doing what investors and artists figured out long ago: they're spreading the work. They're building a portfolio.

A portfolio career for a physician in 2026 means combining income streams, skills, and professional roles so that no single employer, no single RVU target, no single hospital administrator holds all the leverage over your livelihood. It can look like one day of clinical work per week paired with a consulting contract. It can look like a full exit from clinical medicine into a medical affairs role at a biotech company. It can look like medico-legal work done from your home office on Friday afternoons while you keep a part-time hospitalist schedule.

There's no single template. That's the point.

The Portfolio Career Defined

A portfolio career isn't a backup plan. It's a structure. It's built deliberately, the way you'd build any other clinical protocol: assess the situation, identify the options, weigh the tradeoffs, and act.

Most physicians who've made this shift didn't wake up one day and quit. They started by adding one income stream alongside their clinical work. That stream gave them information. It showed them what the market would pay for their expertise, what kinds of work made them feel capable again, and what kind of schedule they actually wanted. Then they adjusted. Some went further non-clinical. Others used the financial cushion to negotiate better clinical terms. A few went fully hybrid and kept it that way permanently.

The portfolio career isn't only for physicians who want to leave medicine. It's also for physicians who want to stay but on better terms. When you have two income streams, your tolerance for a terrible administrator drops. When you have outside clients, you're less dependent on your employer's RVU formula. When you've built something outside the hospital walls, you stop negotiating from desperation.

That shift in leverage changes everything about how you work.

For physicians who do want to exit clinical medicine fully, the portfolio model provides a bridge. You don't have to leap. You can step. You try one role, build one skill set, develop one external relationship. Then you step again. By the time you're ready to walk away from clinical work entirely, you've already got something real on the other side.

The sectors covered in this chapter are not exhaustive. They're the ones where physician expertise translates most directly and where demand in 2026 is strong enough to be worth your attention. If you went through the four-path triage model in Chapter 14 and landed on Lateral Move or Exit, this chapter is where you figure out where you're going.

The Non-Clinical Sectors Hiring MDs in 2026

Health Technology

The health tech sector has been hiring physicians for years, but the role has changed. In the early days, companies mostly wanted doctors to lend credibility to a product. You'd show up at a conference, say something authoritative, and collect a check. That still exists, but it's not the interesting work.

The interesting work in health tech in 2026 is clinical product development, medical direction, and clinical informatics. Companies building AI diagnostic tools, remote patient monitoring platforms, clinical decision support systems, and digital therapeutics need physicians who understand how care actually gets delivered. They need someone who's stood at a nursing station at 2 a.m. and knows exactly why that workflow will fail the moment it hits a real floor.

That's you.

Titles in health tech include Chief Medical Officer, VP of Clinical Affairs, Medical Director, Clinical Product Manager, and Clinical Advisor. The last two don't always require a full-time commitment. Many companies hire physician advisors on retainer or contract terms, which fits the portfolio model well.

What companies want from you isn't your clinical technique. They want your pattern recognition. They want to know what makes a physician trust a tool, what makes a system fail in practice, and what a realistic clinical workflow looks like. You've spent years developing that knowledge. The tech sector will pay well for it.

Entry into health tech often comes through clinical advisory roles, which pay a monthly retainer for a set number of hours. From there, physicians who want more involvement can move toward full-time medical director positions or part-time fractional CMO contracts. Fractional roles are increasingly common. A company that can't afford a full-time CMO will often pay well for eight to twelve hours a month from someone with the right background.

Pharmaceutical and Biotechnology

Pharma and biotech hire physicians across a wide range of functions. The most visible are medical affairs, clinical development, and regulatory affairs. Each has a different day-to-day feel, and knowing which one fits your skills matters before you start applying.

Medical affairs is probably the most common entry point. Medical affairs physicians serve as the scientific and clinical interface between the company and the external medical community. They don't do sales. They engage with key opinion leaders, support medical education programs, respond to unsolicited medical requests, and help ensure the company's clinical communications are accurate and compliant. If you like the intellectual side of medicine, enjoy synthesizing data, and want to work with other clinicians without managing their wellbeing, medical affairs is worth a close look.

Clinical development involves designing and overseeing clinical trials. Physicians in clinical development work with biostatisticians, regulatory teams, and investigators to build trial protocols and monitor safety data. If you trained in research or have a methodological background, this is a natural fit. It's also one of the more demanding roles in terms of hours and travel during active trial phases, so it's less compatible with ongoing clinical work.

Regulatory affairs is a highly specialized function that involves getting drugs and devices approved by the FDA and equivalent international bodies. Many regulatory physicians came out of clinical development or have specific expertise in a therapeutic area relevant to the product. This is a smaller door, but it's open.

Compensation in pharma is generally strong. Total compensation packages often include base salary, annual bonus, equity or stock options, and benefits. The tradeoff is that pharma roles often require more corporate culture navigation than clinical medicine. The politics are different but they're real.

Medical Science Liaison

The MSL role deserves its own section because it's one of the most misunderstood opportunities available to physicians. Many doctors have interacted with MSLs without fully understanding what the role is.

A Medical Science Liaison is a field-based scientific expert employed by a pharmaceutical, biotech, or medical device company. MSLs don't sell. Their job is to build peer-level scientific relationships with physicians and researchers, share clinical data, gather insight about real-world use of therapies, and support medical education.

They're the people who show up to have a genuine scientific conversation, not a sales pitch.

For physicians, the MSL role offers several things that clinical medicine increasingly does not. You set much of your own schedule. You work independently. Your success depends on your knowledge and relationships, not on your RVU count. You're not on call. You're not managing a prior authorization queue at 9 p.m.

The starting point for most physician MSLs is a therapeutic area where they have direct clinical experience. A cardiologist moving into an MSL role will almost always start with a cardiovascular product line. A neurologist will look at neurology-focused companies. Your specialty knowledge is the first credential the company is buying. Your communication skills and scientific fluency are the second.

One thing to understand: MSL roles are field-based, which means travel. Regional roles might require two to three days of travel per week. National roles can be more. If you want location flexibility, this may be worth the tradeoff. If your family situation doesn't support regular travel, the schedule needs to be part of your evaluation from the start.

Physicians who want to keep a small amount of clinical work alongside an MSL role often can. Many companies allow it, provided there's no conflict of interest with the products you support. Get this clarified in writing before you accept an offer.

Consulting

Medical consulting comes in several flavors. Understanding which kind you're pursuing matters because the entry paths, income structures, and day-to-day work are completely different.

Health system and strategy consulting involves working with hospital systems, health plans, or government agencies on organizational, operational, or policy questions. Large consulting firms hire physicians as subject matter experts, particularly in value-based care, population health, utilization management, and health system transformation. If you have an MBA or a strong business background, this door opens faster. If you don't, it's not closed, but you'll need to show you can translate clinical knowledge into business language.

Independent consulting is different. Here, you're not working for a consulting firm. You're building your own client base. Independent physician consultants typically serve one of several markets: healthcare companies needing clinical input on a project basis, law firms needing medical expertise for litigation support, private equity funds doing due diligence on healthcare acquisitions, or technology companies needing a clinical advisor who isn't ready for a full MSL or medical director hire.

Independent consulting takes longer to build than a salaried role, but the ceiling is higher and the autonomy is real. Many physicians start by doing one or two small projects on the side, often through professional connections they already have, and grow the practice from there. The skill set required is less about clinical expertise and more about scoping projects, communicating value to non-clinical clients, and billing for your time without apology.

The medico-legal space overlaps with consulting. Physicians who serve as expert witnesses or independent medical examiners are technically consultants. That sector gets its own discussion below.

Medico-Legal Work

Medico-legal work involves applying your clinical knowledge to legal cases. It includes expert witness testimony, independent medical examinations, medical record review, and case consultation for attorneys.

Expert witness work comes in two main forms. You can work for the plaintiff side, the defense side, or both, depending on your discipline and the cases you choose to accept. Many physicians start with medical record review, which requires no courtroom appearance and can be done entirely in writing. That's a reasonable entry point if the idea of deposition or trial testimony sounds intimidating. You get paid to read records, apply your clinical knowledge, and write a report. The attorney uses that report to understand the case.

As you develop a track record and a reputation, you can move into deposition testimony and eventually trial testimony. Each step adds complexity and typically adds income. Physician expert witnesses with strong credentials and clear communication skills are in demand across specialties.

The medico-legal space has a realistic barrier to entry: your specialty. The cases that need expert testimony are concentrated in specialties with high litigation exposure. Surgeons, OBs, emergency physicians, anesthesiologists, and neurologists tend to find more cases available than, say, a dermatologist or a pediatric subspecialist, though those markets exist too.

One thing that catches physicians off guard in this space is the time gap between accepting a case and getting paid. Medico-legal compensation can be significant, but payment often doesn't come until a case resolves, which can take months or years. Building medico-legal work as your only income stream creates a cash flow problem. It works well as part of a portfolio where other streams cover your monthly expenses.

Structuring a Sustainable Hybrid Life

The goal is a structure that actually works in practice, not just on a spreadsheet.

Many physicians who try to build a portfolio career make the same early mistake. They take on too much too fast. They keep their full-time clinical schedule, add one new commitment, then add another, and end up more exhausted than when they started. The portfolio model done badly just creates a different kind of burnout with a better-looking LinkedIn profile.

The structure that works is built around your Runway Number, which you calculated back in Chapter 13. Your Runway Number tells you what you need to cover your essential expenses. Anything above that number is flexibility. Use that knowledge to sequence your portfolio deliberately.

Start by identifying what you're trading. Most hybrid structures involve trading clinical hours for non-clinical work. If you're currently at 1.0 FTE clinically, you can't add a 20-hour-per-week consulting engagement without something giving way. That something is usually sleep, health, or family time. That's not a portfolio. That's just a different version of the same problem.

A realistic hybrid structure in the early phase might look like this: reduce clinical work to 0.6 or 0.8 FTE while building one external income stream. Use that stream to replace the income lost from the clinical reduction. Once the external stream is stable, assess whether you want to reduce clinical work further or hold at that level.

The sequence matters. You build the external stream while you still have clinical income, so you're not making decisions from a position of financial desperation. You reduce clinical work as the external stream becomes reliable, so you're never without a floor. And you keep evaluating, because the right balance in year one of a portfolio career is rarely the right balance in year three.

Contracts matter in this structure. If you still have a clinical employment contract, check it before you take on any outside work. Many physician employment contracts include broad language about outside employment, moonlighting restrictions, or conflicts of interest. Some of that language is enforceable. Some of it is negotiating bluff. You need an attorney who understands physician employment contracts, not a general practice attorney, to read it with you before you sign anything on the non-clinical side. Chapter 18 covers the CV-to-resume translation and the 12-month planning calendar in detail, so this chapter won't repeat that ground. What matters here is that the legal review happens before you commit.

Tax structure is another piece physicians frequently miss until it costs them money. When you add consulting, MSL retainer work, or expert witness fees to your income, you're typically receiving that income as a self-employed person. That means self-employment tax on top of income tax, quarterly estimated payments, and a set of deductions you may not be using. Setting up a single-member LLC or S-corp for your non-clinical income is worth a conversation with an accountant who works with physicians. The specifics depend on your income level and state, but the conversation should happen early, not at tax time.

Time management in a hybrid life is less complicated than it sounds, but it requires clarity. The physicians who make this work tend to keep their clinical schedule and their non-clinical schedule in separate compartments. They don't take clinical calls during consulting blocks and they don't answer consulting emails during clinic. The boundaries aren't rigid to the point of absurdity, but they're real. If you carry every obligation in your head at all times, you'll be half-present in both roles and fully effective in neither.

The Portfolio Career Menu

Think of this section as a field guide. The sectors above each have different entry requirements, different compensation structures, and different day-to-day realities. Here's a working summary of how to evaluate each one for your situation.

Health Technology is best for physicians who want to stay close to clinical innovation, are comfortable in fast-moving environments, and have a tolerance for some ambiguity about what their role includes on any given week. Entry often starts with advisory contracts. Clinical specialty matters less than your ability to translate clinical realities into product language.

Pharma/Biotech Medical Affairs is best for physicians who like rigorous science, prefer peer-level conversations over administrative ones, and want a structured corporate environment with clear paths to advancement. Your specialty will determine which companies want to talk to you first. Having publications or research experience helps but isn't always required for entry-level medical affairs roles.

MSL is best for physicians who are scientifically strong communicators, comfortable working independently in the field, and willing to travel regularly. You'll need to be honest with yourself about the travel requirement. It's not a paperwork job. If the road suits you, the flexibility and autonomy are real.

Pharma Clinical Development is best for physicians who want to be deeply involved in building the clinical evidence base for a new treatment, have strong methodological knowledge, and are prepared for a demanding schedule during active trials. This is less compatible with ongoing clinical work than the other pharma pathways.

Health System Consulting (Employed) is best for physicians who have an interest in organizational and operational problems, can write and present at a business level, and prefer the security of a salaried role over building an independent practice. Large consulting firms are selective, but physician candidates with subspecialty expertise in areas like oncology, cardiology, or value-based care are in demand.

Independent Consulting is best for physicians who want maximum control over their schedule and client mix, have existing professional relationships they can convert to consulting relationships, and are comfortable with some income variability in the early phase. The ceiling is high and the ceiling belongs to you.

Medico-Legal is best for physicians in high-litigation specialties who have strong written communication skills, a comfort with adversarial processes, and the patience to build a practice over time. It pairs well with clinical work in the early years because the income is irregular and the cases take time.

These aren't ranked. The best option is the one that fits your specialty, your schedule, your financial situation, and what you actually want to do with your time. The physicians who succeed with portfolio careers tend to have one thing in common: they made a real choice. They picked a direction based on honest self-assessment, not on whatever sounded impressive or whatever a colleague happened to mention at a conference. They started somewhere specific and adjusted from there.

Your MD is a clinical credential, but it's also a commercial asset. The market in 2026 has multiple sectors that value that asset and will pay for access to your knowledge, your judgment, and your credibility. What those sectors want from you is not your ability to tolerate a broken system. They want your expertise. That's something you've earned and it belongs to you regardless of which path you choose next.

Where to Start

Pick one sector from the menu above. Just one.

Research three to five companies or firms in that space that are active in your therapeutic area or specialty. Find one person who holds a role similar to what you're targeting. Look at their background. Look at how they got there. You don't need to reach out to them yet. You just need to understand that there is a path, that real physicians are walking it, and that the path has a visible first step.

The next chapter covers the actual mechanics of making the move: converting your CV to a resume, building a network from scratch if you need to, and the 12-month timeline that makes this feel like a plan instead of a wish. For now, the assignment is simpler.

Decide which sector you're taking seriously. Write it down. That decision is the beginning of the structure.

The Transition Blueprint

Most physicians who reach this point have done the hard internal work. They've named what's broken, chosen a path, and started decoupling their identity from the credential. What they haven't done is figure out the mechanics. How do you actually get from here to there? How do you turn a decade of clinical experience into something a non-clinical hiring manager understands? How do you build a professional network when you've spent your entire career inside one institution? How do you keep your finances intact while you're still working a job that's grinding you down?

Those are operational questions. This chapter answers them.

CV to Resume: Translating Clinical Achievement

Your CV is a complete record of your professional existence. Every publication, every conference presentation, every committee you sat on. It can run ten pages or twenty. It proves you are a physician.

A corporate resume does something different. It answers one question: what problems can you solve, and what have you already solved? Hiring managers outside of medicine rarely read past the first page. They don't know what your RVU productivity means. They don't care how many CME hours you've logged. They want to know if you can lead a team, manage a budget, reduce costs, improve a process, or communicate complex information to non-experts.

You can do all of those things. You've been doing them your entire career. The problem is your CV doesn't say that in language they recognize.

The first step is a translation exercise. Go through your CV section by section and ask: what's the business version of this?

Running a clinical service line is department management. Supervising residents and fellows is talent development and coaching. Implementing a new protocol that reduced readmission rates is process improvement with measurable outcomes. Serving on a pharmacy and therapeutics committee is cross-functional collaboration on cost containment. Authoring clinical guidelines is technical writing and subject matter expertise. Handling a patient safety event is crisis management and stakeholder communication.

None of that is a stretch. Every one of those reframes is accurate. You're not lying on your resume. You're translating your real experience into the language your new audience speaks.

The format changes too. A clinical CV lists everything chronologically, starting with medical school. A corporate resume leads with a summary statement at the top, followed by two to three pages maximum of achievement-focused bullet points. Each bullet should start with an action verb and include a result wherever you can quantify it.

Here's the structural difference in practice. Your CV might say: "Faculty, Department of Internal Medicine, 2018-present." Your resume says: "Led a 12-physician faculty team, overseeing clinical quality metrics, resident education, and departmental protocol development for a 400-bed academic center." Same job. Completely different signal.

Quantify everything you can. How many patients did you see per year? How large was the clinical team you supervised? Did you reduce something, improve something, launch something? Even rough numbers work. "Approximately 2,000 patient encounters annually" beats no number at all. "Reduced time-to-discharge by implementing a discharge checklist across a 30-bed unit" is specific enough to be credible without needing a journal citation.

Keep the summary statement short. Three to four lines. Name your specialty, your years of experience, your crossover skills (leadership, data analysis, writing, speaking, clinical operations), and what you're moving toward. If you're going into pharma medical affairs, say so. If you're targeting health tech, say so. The summary tells the reader immediately whether your profile fits their need.

Drop the medical jargon in the body of the resume. "Board-certified" is fine. "Proficient in ICD-10 coding" means nothing to a tech recruiter. "Reduced prior authorization denials by 30% through payer negotiations and documentation process redesign" means a lot, because it shows you understand the intersection of clinical and business.

Keep a separate master file with everything on it. Your resume is a curated selection from that master file, not a permanent document. Tailor it for each application. The resume you send to a pharmaceutical company for a Medical Science Liaison role looks different from the one you send to a health insurance company for a Medical Director role. The core is the same. The emphasis shifts.

One more thing about the CV-to-resume translation. Include a skills section. Physicians undersell their technical skills because they assume everyone can do what they do. Put in clinical decision-making, EHR systems, protocol development, literature review, data interpretation, patient safety, regulatory compliance, quality improvement methodology, public speaking, and medical writing if it applies. These are real skills. Name them explicitly.

Networking Without an Existing Network

Most physicians have a professional network that's almost entirely clinical. Colleagues in your specialty, maybe a handful of people from residency, some attendings you still respect. That network can't get you a pharma job or a health tech role or a consulting engagement. It wasn't built for that.

Building a non-clinical network feels awkward, especially when you've been inside a single institution for years. You're not a natural networker. Nobody trained you to be. Medicine selected for people who kept their head down, worked hard, and let results speak for them.

The results don't speak loudly enough in a world where you don't have a track record yet. The network does.

Start with LinkedIn. Optimize your profile before you do anything else. Your headline should say more than your title. "Internal Medicine Physician" doesn't differentiate you. "Physician Leader | Clinical Operations | Pharma Transition | Healthcare Consulting" tells someone what you offer and what you're looking for. Update your About section to reflect where you're headed, not just where you've been. Use the same language you put in your resume summary.

Then start connecting with people who are already doing what you want to do. Search for physicians in non-clinical roles. Search for Medical Science Liaisons, Chief Medical Officers at tech companies, physician consultants, medical affairs professionals. Connect with a short, specific message. Don't ask for a job. Ask for 20 minutes of their time to learn how they made the transition.

Most people who've successfully crossed over are willing to talk. They remember what it felt like to not know how the crossing worked. A short message that says "I'm a hospitalist with 12 years of experience considering a move into medical affairs. I'd love 20 minutes to learn how you approached the transition" gets responses. A generic "I'd like to connect" gets ignored.

Set a weekly target. Five new connections per week. Two informational interview requests per week. That's a manageable pace that compounds over 12 months into a real network.

Informational interviews are the most underused tool in physician career transitions. They're conversations, not job interviews. The goal is to understand how someone else got to where they are, what their day actually looks like, what skills matter, what they wish they'd known, and whether they'd be willing to refer you to someone else when the time comes.

Keep notes after each conversation. What did you learn? What's the next step this person suggested? Who did they mention that you should talk to? Over time you'll start to see patterns. You'll hear the same names, the same certifications, the same companies repeatedly. That tells you where to focus.

Beyond LinkedIn, look at physician-specific communities that bridge clinical and non-clinical worlds. Organizations like the American College of Healthcare Executives, the Physician Executive MBA programs, and specialty-specific groups often host events and have listservs where physicians in transition share leads and introductions. Local healthcare conferences that bring together executives, investors, and operators are worth attending even once. You're not going to get hired at a conference. But you'll meet people, exchange contact information, and have a reason to follow up.

Don't underestimate the value of the physicians you already know. Your current colleagues may have spouses, partners, or former classmates who work in pharma, health tech, or consulting. They may have left medicine themselves and built connections they'd share. You don't need to announce that you're leaving. A simple "I've been exploring some adjacent opportunities and I'm curious if you know anyone who works in medical affairs or health technology" opens doors without requiring a full disclosure conversation.

Your clinical expertise is genuinely valuable to people outside medicine. You know things that non-physicians spend years trying to understand. How physicians make decisions. How hospital systems work. What matters to patients. Why a drug gets adopted or ignored. Why a technology that looks good on paper fails at the point of care. People will pay for that knowledge. They'll hire for it. And they'll refer others to you once you've shown them what you bring.

The 12-Month Phase-Out Plan

The 12-month timeline isn't a rigid contract. It's a framework. Some transitions move faster. Some take 18 months. What matters is having a structure so you're not just drifting and hoping something changes. Hope is not a plan.

Months 1 through 3: Foundations

This phase is about getting your house in order before you start knocking on doors.

Calculate your Runway Number if you haven't already. As covered in Chapter 13, that number tells you how many months of financial stability you have if your income stopped today. If you don't know that number, every career decision you make is a guess. Month one, you run those numbers.

Pull your current employment contract and read it. Look specifically at the non-compete clause. How many miles does it cover? How many months? Does it apply to non-clinical work? Many non-competes are written broadly but enforced narrowly. Knowing exactly what yours says before you start exploring options prevents surprises later. If your contract is confusing, a healthcare attorney can review it for a few hundred dollars. That's money well spent.

Update your CV during this phase. Start the translation exercise described earlier. Get a draft resume done. It doesn't have to be perfect yet, but having a current draft ready means you're not scrambling later.

Start your LinkedIn optimization. Update your headline and About section. Add a professional photo if you don't have one. Begin connecting with people in the spaces you're exploring.

Also in months one through three: get clear on your target. Refer back to Chapter 17 and the non-clinical sectors. Which one fits your skills, your schedule needs, and your financial requirements? Narrowing to two or three realistic targets at this stage focuses everything that comes next.

Months 4 through 6: Skill Building and Visibility

This phase is about filling gaps and showing up in new spaces.

What certifications or credentials would strengthen your case for the roles you're targeting? Medical affairs roles often value a Medical Science Liaison certification course. Health tech companies value product thinking, which you can start developing through free resources and short courses. Consulting work values structured communication and financial literacy. None of these take years to develop. But a few months of deliberate investment makes your resume sharper and gives you credibility in conversations.

Run your informational interviews in earnest during this phase. Aim for two per week. Take notes. Follow up. Say thank you within 24 hours. The people you talk to in months four through six become references and referrers in months nine through twelve.

Consider writing. A LinkedIn article about your perspective on a clinical problem that the industry is trying to solve gets you visibility in communities where hiring managers live. You don't have to write for publication. A thoughtful 600-word post once a week demonstrates you can communicate, that you understand the intersection of clinical and business, and that you're showing up consistently. That matters.

If your target is pharma or biotech, look at whether there are part-time or consulting opportunities where you can start building a track record while still employed. Some companies are willing to pay physicians for advisory work, consulting calls, or market research on a per-project basis. Even one small paid engagement establishes that you're someone who crosses over successfully.

Months 7 through 9: Applications and Interviews

Now you have a network, a polished resume, and targeted knowledge of your sectors. It's time to apply.

Physician job boards serve clinical roles. For non-clinical work, use LinkedIn, company career pages, and referrals from your informational interview network. A referral from someone inside the company dramatically increases the odds your resume gets a real read. That's why the network work in months four through six pays off here.

Tailor your application materials for each role. The resume you send to a pharmaceutical medical affairs team emphasizes your knowledge of disease states, clinical trial interpretation, and physician relationships. The resume you send to a healthcare consulting firm emphasizes your analytical skills, protocol development experience, and ability to communicate complex information clearly. Same background, different emphasis.

Prepare for interviews differently than you prepared for medical interviews. Corporate interviews lean heavily on behavioral questions. "Tell me about a time when you had to influence people without direct authority." "Describe a situation where you had to manage a conflict between two stakeholders." "Walk me through how you'd approach a new market research project." These questions pull from clinical experience. Your answer about navigating a disagreement with hospital administration over staffing levels is a perfect answer to a question about managing stakeholder conflict. Practice converting your clinical stories into behavioral interview answers before the first call.

Negotiate. Physicians are historically bad at this. Corporate roles often have room for base salary movement, bonus structure, sign-on bonuses, remote work provisions, and start date flexibility. Research salary ranges before any offer conversation. Sites that aggregate compensation by role and experience level can give you a benchmark.

Know the number you need, know the number you want, and don't accept the first offer without at least one counteroffer. This is normal in corporate hiring. It won't cost you the offer.

Months 10 through 12: Execution and Exit

You've accepted an offer, or you're close. Now you manage the exit.

Review your contract one more time, specifically the notice provisions. Most physician contracts require 60 to 90 days notice. Some require more. Build that into your timeline. Accepting an offer and then discovering your contract requires four months notice creates a problem.

Have the resignation conversation with your employer after the offer letter is signed and countersigned. Not before. Write a formal resignation letter that is professional and brief. It doesn't need to explain your reasons in detail. It needs to give your notice period, confirm your last day, and express that you'll support a smooth transition. Keep the tone neutral even if the relationship was bad.

Plan your transition of care deliberately. Your patients deserve continuity. Prepare a transition summary for your panel. Give your team enough lead time to redistribute your patient load. Do this with care, because your reputation in the clinical community is something you may need to leverage later, even if you're leaving it.

Managing the Transition Period

The months between deciding to leave and actually leaving are among the hardest in this process. You're still doing the job that's draining you while building a new life on the side. Your colleagues may not know. Your employer may not know. You're holding two versions of your career simultaneously.

That dual reality is exhausting. Give yourself permission for it to be exhausting. It won't last forever. It lasts exactly as long as the transition period.

A few things make it more manageable.

Keep the new work contained. If you're doing informational interviews and resume work and skill building during the transition, do it outside of your clinical hours. Don't do it on your employer's time or systems. This protects you legally, ethically, and practically. It also protects your concentration during patient care, which is the one place you can't afford to be distracted.

Don't tell your employer before you're ready. You don't owe them advance warning beyond your contractual notice period. Many physicians feel obligated to be transparent with administration, to give extra time, to soften the departure in every possible way. That instinct comes from years of being the good colleague, the reliable one, the one who doesn't rock the boat. Your employer is not applying the same standard to you. They will replace you before you're out the door. Be professional. Follow your contract. You don't owe more than that.

Watch the finances closely during this period. If you have significant signing bonuses that you'd need to repay if you leave before a certain date, factor that into your exit timing. If your health insurance is tied to your current employment, know exactly when it ends and when your new coverage begins. COBRA exists, but it's expensive. Gap coverage matters.

Tell the people who need to know. Your spouse or partner needs to know you're in transition because the household finances and schedule are both affected. A mentor you trust may be worth telling because they can give you perspective when the transition feels slow. Your colleagues don't need to know until you're ready, and your institution definitely doesn't need to know before you hand in your resignation.

There will be a moment, probably somewhere in months eight through ten, when you feel simultaneously exhausted and alive. You're tired from carrying two full professional lives. You're energized because the new one is actually taking shape. That feeling is a good sign. It means the transition is real, not just theoretical.

The transition from clinical medicine to a non-clinical role doesn't require starting over from scratch. You're not a new graduate trying to prove yourself with no track record. You're a physician with deep expertise, strong analytical skills, and lived experience inside the system that healthcare companies are trying to understand and sell into. That's worth something. In some contexts, it's worth considerably more than you've been paid for it.

The blueprint is here. The 12-month frame gives you a structure. The CV translation gives you a document that opens doors. The networking strategy gives you access. The exit planning gives you a clean departure. What comes after that is covered in the next chapter.

For now, the question is simpler: what's your month one action?

Your Starting Checklist

These are the six things to do in your first 30 days, in order:

1. Calculate your Runway Number. Pull your last three months of bank and credit card statements. Know your monthly expenses cold.

2. Read your employment contract. Write down your non-compete radius, duration, and scope. Write down your notice period. Keep that paper.

3. Draft your resume using the CV translation process in this chapter. Get one version done even if it's not perfect.

4. Optimize your LinkedIn profile. Update your headline, your About section, and your photo.

5. Identify your two to three target non-clinical sectors from Chapter 17.

6. Schedule your first two informational interviews. Reach out this week.

Month one isn't about having everything figured out. It's about having the foundations in place so that months two through twelve can actually move.

The Regenerated Physician

You made it through the hardest part. You diagnosed the system. You named the exploitation. You built a runway, ran your triage, and started moving toward something that actually fits your life. Whether you stayed and restructured, pivoted sideways, or walked out the door entirely, you did the work most physicians are too scared or too exhausted to attempt.

But here's what nobody tells you about recovery: it doesn't end when the acute crisis ends.

The physician who burned through everything to get here is not the same person who will carry this forward. Regeneration isn't a one-time event. It's a practice. And like any clinical skill, it degrades without upkeep. The systems that broke you in the first place are still out there. The pressure to over-give, over-produce, and under-protect yourself didn't disappear when you renegotiated your contract or left your health system. It lives in your habits, your reflexes, and sometimes your own head.

This chapter is about keeping what you've built. Protecting the changes you made. Staying connected to the reasons you made them. And continuing to act like someone who owns their career rather than someone who just survived one.

Long-Term Boundary Audits

Boundaries erode. That's not a character flaw. It's physics. When you set a limit and the immediate pressure backs off, it gets easier to let things slide a little. Then a little more. Six months from now, you might look up and realize you're answering messages at 10 p.m. again. Your protected Fridays got eaten by "just this one urgent consult." Your clinical hours crept back up when the practice manager asked for a favor.

This is normal. It's also preventable with one simple habit: the scheduled boundary audit.

Schedule a quarterly review of your working conditions. Put it on the calendar like a board meeting, because it is one. You're the board. Your life is the company. The review doesn't have to take long, but it has to be honest.

Start with time. Track your actual hours for two weeks before the audit, not what your schedule says, but what you actually worked. Include charting time, inbox time, administrative tasks you took home, and calls you answered outside your agreed hours. If that number has drifted upward since the last audit, you need to know by how much and why.

Then look at your inbox metrics. How long does it take you to clear messages on a typical day? Are you still getting patient portal messages at volume you can't handle without spilling into personal time? If you negotiated inbox boundaries and they've dissolved, that's information. It tells you the original agreement needs reinforcement, a formal conversation, or structural support like a triage nurse or message protocol.

Next, look at your no-rate. How often did you say no to committee work, extra shifts, admin tasks, or peer requests last quarter? If the answer is "not much," ask yourself whether you genuinely chose those commitments or whether you defaulted back into automatic compliance. There's a difference between adding something that genuinely serves you and adding something because you didn't have the energy to push back.

Finally, look at your physical state. Are you sleeping? Eating at reasonable hours? Moving your body with any regularity? These aren't wellness lecture checklist items. They're operational indicators. When they tank, output quality and decision-making follow. A physician running on poor sleep and skipped lunches isn't a resilient professional. That person is burning credit they'll have to repay later.

Do this review four times a year. Write it down. Compare it to the previous quarter. If something has slipped, address it before it compounds. The physicians who sustain recovery are the ones who treat boundary maintenance as ongoing infrastructure work, not a one-time installation.

Measuring the New Life

Most physicians are excellent at measuring clinical outcomes. You know your A1C panels, your patient panel size, your RVU counts, your Press Ganey scores. What many physicians have never done is build a personal measurement system for their own life.

That changes now.

Pick three to five metrics that matter to you. These are yours, so they should reflect what you actually care about, not what your employer cares about or what you think you should care about. Some physicians measure sleep hours per week. Some track the number of mornings they don't dread going in. Some measure time with family, hours spent on creative work, books read, or weeks without a Sunday-evening spiral of dread.

Whatever your metrics are, write them down and check them monthly. You're looking for trends, not perfection. You're asking: is my life moving in the direction I chose, or is it drifting back toward a pattern I deliberately left?

The point of measurement isn't to hold yourself to some ideal standard. It's to stay honest. Physicians are good at telling themselves stories when the evidence doesn't match. "It's just this month." "Things will settle down after Q3." "I'm managing fine." Measurement cuts through the story. The number either moved or it didn't.

Build your personal dashboard using whatever format works for you. A notebook. A spreadsheet. A note in your phone. It doesn't need to be elaborate. It just needs to exist and be used. Monthly check-ins with your own data are more useful than annual performance reviews written by someone who doesn't know what your career costs you.

One specific metric worth tracking is your clinical load relative to your stated limit. If you transitioned to a reduced clinical schedule, track the actual hours quarterly and flag any upward creep. Scope expansion is the most common way physicians who restructured their work find themselves back at unsustainable volume twelve months later. The slope is always gradual. Measurement catches it while it's still fixable.

Another metric worth keeping: financial runway. As discussed in Chapter 13, your Runway Number is the months of expenses your liquid savings can cover without any income. Track this quarterly too. A growing runway means more options and more leverage. A shrinking runway means you're vulnerable. Know which direction it's moving.

Staying Connected to Purpose

One of the risks of a major career restructure is losing the thread back to why you became a physician in the first place. When you're in crisis mode, survival is the goal. Once you're out of crisis, there's sometimes a strange flatness. You removed the thing that was breaking you, but you haven't yet filled that space with something that energizes you. That transition period can feel disorienting.

You don't need to feel passion every day. That's not how meaningful work functions for most people. But you do need periodic contact with the reason you chose this field, whatever version of that reason still feels true.

For some physicians, that contact comes through direct patient care. Even if you've moved primarily into consulting, advisory work, or a portfolio career, maintaining a small amount of clinical work can anchor the sense of purpose that pulled you into medicine. This isn't mandatory. For some people, a clean break is healthier. But if you find yourself missing the direct clinical relationship, a small amount of carefully protected clinical time can serve a real function.

For others, purpose reconnects through teaching or mentorship. If you're further along in your career, there are residents and early-career physicians navigating the same system that nearly broke you. Your hard-won perspective has value. Informal mentorship, whether that's a regular check-in with a younger colleague or a more structured advisor role, keeps you engaged with the next generation of physicians without requiring you to re-enter the most toxic parts of the system.

Some physicians find purpose through advocacy. The work in Chapter 15 on collective action isn't only for people still embedded in health systems. Former physicians, portfolio physicians, and hybrid-career physicians carry credibility in policy discussions that pure administrators lack. If the systemic failures that drove your exit still anger you, that anger is information. It can fuel useful work.

The key is making purpose contact intentional. When you're burned out, purpose gets buried under survival. When you're recovering, it can get bypassed because you're busy rebuilding. Don't wait until you feel the familiar emptiness before you check in on it. Make it a scheduled practice, the same way you scheduled your boundary audit.

Once a quarter, ask yourself: what part of my current work feels most worth doing? What am I doing because I chose it, and what am I doing by default? Is there something I keep putting off that would actually reconnect me to what matters? Those questions aren't soft. They're operational. The answers tell you where to invest and where to scale back.

The Ongoing Practice of Agency

Agency isn't something you achieve and then have forever. It's something you exercise. Like any muscle, it weakens without use. The physicians who stay regenerated are the ones who keep making active choices about their careers rather than sliding back into passive compliance.

The healthcare system hasn't fixed itself while you were doing this work. Corporate capture is still happening. Prior authorization burdens are still rising. The pressure to produce at unsustainable rates is still built into most employment models. You've built a buffer against those forces. That buffer requires maintenance.

What does active agency look like in practice?

It looks like reviewing your contract every year, even if you don't plan to renegotiate. Know what it says. Know when key clauses expire. Know whether the compensation model has shifted in ways that disadvantage you. A physician who knows their contract can act on what they find. A physician who hasn't read it since signing is flying blind.

It looks like keeping your professional network alive outside your current employer. This isn't about disloyalty. It's about options. Physicians with strong external networks have leverage. They have somewhere to go if conditions deteriorate.

They hear about opportunities before they're posted publicly. If your network went dormant while you were in survival mode, revive it. One meaningful professional conversation per month is enough to keep it functional.

It looks like staying current on your non-clinical skills. If you built a portfolio career or a hybrid model, those skills need ongoing development just like clinical competency. Medical advisory roles, consulting engagements, pharma or tech work, medical-legal practice, each of these has its own professional landscape that evolves. Set aside time to stay current. Read the trade press in your non-clinical area. Attend one non-clinical conference per year. Keep developing expertise that doesn't depend on your clinical license.

It looks like revisiting your four-path triage every year. As we laid out in Chapter 14, the paths are Stay/Repair, Stay/Shrink, Lateral Move, and Exit. Your current path was the right choice at the time you made it. A year from now, the situation will be different. Maybe your health system was acquired. Maybe a new non-clinical opportunity appeared. Maybe you've healed enough to consider returning to a modified clinical role you previously left. The triage isn't a one-time assessment. Run it annually and let the result inform your next move.

Agency also means protecting your mental health with the same rigor you protected your clinical skills. If you sought support while working through the crisis chapters of this book, don't drop that support the moment things stabilize. Stability is when ongoing support is most cost-effective, because you're not in crisis, you're doing maintenance. The physicians who wait until they're back at rock bottom before seeking help are reinvesting crisis costs that could have been avoided.

There's a pattern that shows up across medicine: a physician hits a wall, makes changes, feels better, and gradually relaxes every protective habit they built during the hard season. Within a year or two, they're back where they started, sometimes worse, because now they've depleted reserves that haven't fully recovered. The regenerated physician breaks that cycle by refusing to treat recovery as a destination.

Think of it like monitoring a chronic condition. You don't stop tracking once the numbers improve. You maintain the protocol that produced the improvement. The protocol is your boundary audit, your personal dashboard, your annual contract review, your maintained network, your non-clinical skill development, and your quarterly purpose check-in. Together, they function as a maintenance regimen for a career and a life that's finally working.

The Physician You Are Now

The version of you that opened this book is not the version that's closing it.

You know what burnout actually is, the Maslach Triad, moral injury, and the difference between individual failure and structural design. You know how corporate capture operates and what prior authorization costs you personally. You've mapped your inbox burden, looked at your contract with clear eyes, and calculated a Runway Number. You've run your triage, made a path decision, and built a transition plan or at least started one.

That knowledge doesn't expire. It compounds. Every time you catch an encroaching boundary and address it, every time you review your contract before a problem surfaces, every time you say no to a committee that would drain you for nothing, you're doing something most of your colleagues never learned to do.

This isn't about being a difficult employee or an unhelpful colleague. It's about being a physician with enough energy, clarity, and stability to actually do good work over the long arc of a career. The physicians who protect themselves aren't the ones who care less. They're often the ones who care enough to stay in it for decades rather than flaming out in their forties.

The system will keep testing your limits. Administrators will ask for more. Patients will push past boundaries you've set. New technology will promise to solve old problems while creating new forms of invisible labor. None of that has changed.

What's changed is you.

You know the patterns now. You know how drift starts. You know what the early warning signs feel like when the load is becoming unsustainable. You have a language for what was happening to you and a set of tools to respond before it becomes a crisis again.

Three things to carry from here:

First, schedule your quarterly boundary audit before you finish reading this chapter. Put a recurring reminder in your calendar. Name it whatever you want. Just make sure it exists.

Second, build your personal dashboard this week. Choose three metrics that tell you honestly whether your life is moving in the direction you chose. Set a monthly date to check them.

Third, revisit your triage one year from today. Set a calendar reminder now. The question isn't whether your choice was right when you made it. The question is whether it's still right and whether a better option has appeared since.

You came into this book burning at both ends. That was never sustainable, and it was never your fault. The forces that produced that exhaustion were deliberate, structural, and well-funded. You have now spent time understanding those forces and building something that doesn't collapse under them.

Keep building. Keep auditing. Keep choosing.

That's what a regenerated physician does.

Your Degree Is a Tool, Not a Life Sentence

You made it through the whole book. That means something. It means you're still fighting, still thinking, still refusing to just accept the version of medicine that's been handed to you. That refusal is the whole point.

This isn't a chapter about wrapping things up neatly. Medicine doesn't work that way, and neither does the kind of change this book is asking you to consider. What this chapter is about is making sure you leave with a clear head, a real plan, and the firm understanding that your MD belongs to you. The system didn't give it to you. A corporation didn't give it to you. You earned it. And you can use it however you decide.

The Reframe That Changes Everything

Here's what most physicians were never told: your degree is a credential, not a covenant.

That might sound obvious when you read it. It doesn't feel obvious when you're living inside a system that spent a decade and a half training you to believe otherwise. Medical school doesn't just teach anatomy and pharmacology. It teaches identity. It teaches you that being a physician is who you are, not what you do. And once that idea is inside you, the system uses it to extract everything it can.

The hospitals know you'll absorb the impossible inbox load because you're "dedicated to your patients." The RVU model works because you'll push through exhaustion before you'll let productivity slide. Prior authorization is a solvable problem for hospital administrators, but they let physicians carry it because physicians will carry it. The entire machinery of corporate medicine runs on the energy of people who believe that stopping means they've failed someone.

That belief is the leverage point. And this book has been about dismantling it.

When you see your degree as a credential instead of a covenant, the math changes. A credential is a tool. A tool gets used strategically. You pick it up when it serves you and set it down when it doesn't. You use it in different contexts. You combine it with other skills. You make decisions about how and where and for how long it gets applied. Tools don't have loyalty. They serve the person holding them.

Your MD opens doors in clinical medicine, yes. It also opens doors in pharmaceutical consulting, health technology, medical-legal work, direct primary care, policy, medical education, insurance utilization review, life sciences, venture capital, digital health startups, and a dozen other fields covered in Chapter 17. The degree is the same degree in every one of those contexts. What changes is how you choose to use it.

This reframe doesn't mean abandoning patients. It doesn't mean walking away from everything that drew you to medicine. It means reclaiming the right to decide how you show up, for how long, and on what terms. A physician who has sovereignty over their career is a better physician, a more present colleague, a healthier person. Depletion doesn't serve anyone, and choosing to protect yourself isn't selfishness. It's strategy.

The system wants you to believe the two things can't coexist: caring deeply about patients and setting firm limits on what you'll absorb. They can. They must. And the physicians who have figured that out are still practicing medicine, still doing meaningful work, and not burning up in the process.

What the Burned-Out Physician Deserves

You deserve an honest accounting of what happened to you.

You went into medicine with real skill and genuine motivation. You completed a training process that strips sleep, social connection, and self-determination for years at a stretch. You emerged with significant debt, significant expertise, and a set of expectations about what medicine would look like. Then you hit the reality: the RVU treadmill, the inbox that runs past midnight, the prior auth denials, the corporate scripts, the administrators who've never seen a patient telling you how to practice. The gap between what you were promised and what you got is real. It's documented. It's not in your head.

As we covered in the early chapters of this book, the Maslach Triad describes burnout as exhaustion, depersonalization, and reduced personal accomplishment. But what's happening to most physicians goes beyond the clinical definition. It's moral injury. It's the wound that comes from being forced, over and over, to act against your own professional judgment. To deny the scan you know the patient needs. To rush the appointment you know needs more time. To sign off on decisions you didn't make and don't agree with. That's not just stress. It's a specific kind of damage.

And the system's answer to that damage has been wellness programs. Mindfulness sessions. Resilience workshops. In some cases, literally coloring books. The message underneath all of it is that the problem lives inside you and that you need to fix your reaction rather than change your situation. That message is false. The research is clear that physician distress is a structural problem, driven by workload, administrative burden, loss of autonomy, and institutional culture. Individual coping skills don't fix structural failures.

You deserve to hear that clearly and without softening. The wellness-lecture response to a systemic crisis isn't just insufficient. It's a form of gaslighting. It redirects your energy toward adjusting your mindset while the actual conditions remain unchanged.

What you also deserve is a clear understanding of your options. Not the options a burned-out, identity-fused physician sees at 11 p.m. after a brutal call week (stay and suffer, or quit and lose everything), but the actual range of options that exists when you step back and look at the whole board.

The Four-Path Burnout Triage Model from Chapter 14 maps that range. Stay/Repair means staying in clinical medicine but rebuilding the conditions of your work, negotiating better terms, eliminating the tasks that aren't yours to carry, and enforcing real limits. Stay/Shrink means reducing your clinical footprint to a sustainable size while adding other income streams so that the system doesn't have total control over your financial life. Lateral Move means staying in medicine but shifting your role, moving into administration, education, consulting, or a hybrid model that uses your clinical training without putting you back in the same unsustainable position. Exit means leaving clinical medicine for a portfolio career that may include some medical work and may not, built on your terms, using your credential in sectors that value it.

All four paths are legitimate. None of them is failure. The path that fits your life, your finances, your health, and your goals is the right path. No one else gets to make that determination.

You also deserve financial clarity. The Runway Number from Chapter 13 is the foundation of every real decision you can make. Without knowing your personal financial floor, you can't evaluate any path clearly. Physicians often stay in destructive situations because they haven't done the math. When they do the math, they frequently discover they have more options than they thought. That number changes what's possible.

The Toolkit: Your Operational Next Steps

Everything in this book connects to one of six tools in the appendices. These aren't bonuses. They're the operational infrastructure that turns the concepts in each chapter into actual decisions and actual changes.

Burnout Vital Signs Checklist

The self-diagnostic at the back of this book gives you a concrete way to measure where you are right now. Burnout doesn't always announce itself clearly. More often it shows up as irritability that seems out of proportion, a growing inability to care about outcomes you used to care about, physical fatigue that sleep doesn't fix, and a creeping sense that nothing you do actually matters. The checklist puts specific questions to each dimension of the Maslach Triad and adds a moral injury index so you can distinguish between exhaustion and the specific weight of being forced to act against your values.

Use it now. Use it again in 90 days. If you're using the Stay/Repair path, use it as a quarterly check to measure whether your interventions are working. If your scores aren't improving after six months of genuine effort, that's data. It means the conditions around you haven't changed enough to support your recovery, and it's time to reconsider your path.

Contract Red Flag Checklist

If you're staying in clinical medicine, renegotiating your contract, or considering a new position, this checklist is non-negotiable before you sign anything. Chapter 9 walked through the anatomy of a predatory contract: the noncompete clauses that limit your mobility for years after you leave, the tail coverage provisions that can cost you tens of thousands of dollars, the APP oversight requirements buried in the fine print, and the call traps that turn a reasonable schedule into something unsustainable.

The checklist pulls every one of those red flags into a single review document. Walk through it with a healthcare attorney before you sign. The cost of that consultation is a fraction of the cost of a bad contract.

Boundary Scripts

Chapter 11 established that boundaries are medical equipment. They protect your capacity to practice. The scripts in the appendix give you the exact verbal and written language to use when administrators push new responsibilities on you, when committees expect your unpaid attendance, when the inbox grows beyond what's clinically necessary, and when colleagues or employers use guilt as a management tool.

Scripts matter because in high-pressure moments, most people revert to old patterns. Having the language already worked out means you don't have to generate it while also managing your response to pressure. You can use the script, stay calm, and hold the position. Practice the scripts before you need them. The ones that feel most uncomfortable to say are usually the ones you need most.

Financial Freedom Worksheet

This is the Runway Number calculator. It walks you through your current monthly fixed costs, your current income, your liquid assets, your debt obligations, and the minimum monthly income you'd need from a new arrangement to cover your floor. It also includes a section for calculating what a 20% clinical reduction would cost you versus what it would save you in overhead, malpractice, and health costs.

Most physicians who complete this worksheet are surprised. Either they discover they're closer to financial flexibility than they thought, or they identify specific costs that are creating unnecessary vulnerability, costs that can be addressed before any career decision happens. Either outcome is useful.

If the worksheet reveals you're more exposed than you realized, that's not a reason to stay stuck. It's a reason to build the runway first. The 12-Month Transition Calendar tells you exactly how to do that.

Portfolio Career Menu

Chapter 17 covered the sectors hiring MDs in 2026: health technology, pharmaceutical medical affairs, medical science liaison roles, medical-legal consulting, utilization review, insurance medical directorates, direct primary care, concierge medicine, health policy, life sciences, medical writing, and executive health. The Portfolio Career Menu in the appendix is a curated directory that maps each sector to the clinical specialties most in demand, typical compensation ranges, the credentials or training that help with entry, and the realistic timeline from initial outreach to first paid engagement.

The menu is designed to be a starting point for research, not a guarantee. Compensation in any non-clinical sector varies by experience, geography, employer, and negotiation. Use it to identify two or three sectors that match your specialty and interests, then move to informational interviews with physicians already working in those areas. The conversations you have with actual people doing this work will tell you more than any list.

The 12-Month Transition Calendar

This is the operational timeline. It assumes you're starting from a full clinical load and moves you through 12 months of structured action, regardless of which path you're taking. The calendar divides into four quarters.

Quarter one is the foundation quarter. You complete the Burnout Vital Signs Checklist, calculate your Runway Number, identify your target path from the triage model, and begin building the financial buffer that gives you genuine options. If you're targeting a non-clinical transition, you update your LinkedIn profile, identify your target sectors, and schedule your first three informational interviews.

Quarter two is the skill-building and network quarter. If you're staying in clinical medicine and pursuing Stay/Repair, you identify the two or three specific working conditions you need to change and begin the formal negotiation process. If you're transitioning, you begin any targeted training or certification your target sector requires, attend your first sector-specific event, and make direct contact with at least five physicians already working in your target area.

Quarter three is the test-and-commit quarter. If you're Stay/Shrink, this is where you implement the reduced schedule. If you're in transition, this is where you pursue your first paid non-clinical engagement, whether that's a consulting project, an advisory role, a locum assignment that funds the transition, or a part-time role in a new sector. By the end of quarter three, you should have evidence about whether your target path is viable.

Quarter four is the stabilization quarter. You've made your move or made your decision to stay and modify. Now you build the systems that protect what you've built. You schedule your next Burnout Vital Signs review. You do a contract review if you're staying. You audit your financial position against your Runway Number. You identify one relationship in your new network to maintain and deepen.

Twelve months isn't magic. Some transitions take longer. Some happen faster. The calendar is a scaffold, not a contract. Use it to maintain momentum when the day-to-day pressure of clinical work makes it easy to defer decisions indefinitely.

Permission Granted

The system counted on you never reaching this page.

It counted on the exhaustion doing its job: keeping your head down, keeping you too tired to plan, keeping you financially dependent enough that the cost of changing felt higher than the cost of staying. It counted on the identity fusion doing the rest, making you feel that questioning the terms of your practice was the same as betraying your patients, betraying medicine, betraying the version of yourself that survived training.

You've read the data. You've seen the analysis. You know that physician burnout is not a character flaw or a resilience failure. It's a predictable output of a system that extracts more than it gives back, that replaced the physician-patient relationship with a production quota, that buried clinical judgment under administrative process, and that used a calling-culture mythology to justify paying for sacrifice with meaning instead of money and autonomy.

You know what moral injury is and why it's different from stress. You know how private equity reshaped the employment landscape. You know what a predatory contract looks like before you sign it. You know what the gender attrition data reveals about structural failure. You know what the Runway Number is and why calculating it changes the conversation. You know the four paths. You know the toolkit.

Now comes the part that's actually hardest: using what you know.

That's not a platitude. Physicians are among the highest-functioning people in any professional category, and the barrier to acting on this knowledge isn't intelligence. The barrier is a combination of legitimate financial pressure, deep identity investment, real fear about what change looks like, and an institutional culture that punishes people who step out of line. Those are real obstacles. This book doesn't minimize any of them.

What this book has tried to do, from the first page to this one, is give you something more powerful than inspiration. Inspiration fades. Data, frameworks, checklists, scripts, and a clear understanding of what's actually happening to you and why, that's what holds up when the pressure is back on and the default is to just keep absorbing.

Your degree belongs to you. It always has. The system borrowed it. It used the years of your training and the depth of your commitment to build revenue models that extract value from your skill while giving you less and less control over how that skill gets applied. That arrangement is renegotiable. The terms are not permanent. The contract with corporate medicine is not the same contract you signed when you chose this field.

You don't have to leave to reclaim your career. Some of you will stay in clinical medicine and fight for better conditions, better contracts, and a practice that actually sustains you. Some of you will shrink your clinical footprint and build the financial independence that removes the coercion from the equation. Some of you will shift sideways into roles that use your training in different ways. Some of you will exit and build something new.

All of those are good outcomes if they're made with clear eyes, solid information, and genuine agency.

The physicians who break completely aren't the ones who made hard choices. They're the ones who kept deferring the choice because the system made deferral feel safer than decision. Deferral is the system's best tool. Don't let it work.

Pick up your toolkit. Run your Runway Number. Work through the triage model. Take the first step on the calendar. Talk to a physician who's already doing what you're considering. Review your contract with someone who understands what they're looking at. Enforce the first limit that needs enforcing.

That's the whole playbook. It's not complicated. It's just hard, which is a different thing entirely.

You went into medicine because you're capable of doing hard things. You proved that over and over through training, through licensing, through clinical decisions that required real skill under real pressure. The work of reclaiming your career is hard in a different way. It requires honesty about what's not working, willingness to break with an identity that's served you and constrained you at the same time, and the patience to build something sustainable rather than just surviving the next shift.

You can do that. The evidence is in how far you've read.

The degree is yours. Use it.

About the Author

About the Author

Jonathan D. Block, MD, MBA, MLS, MPH, CPE is a physician, executive, consultant, and founder of Pierhead Lighthouse, a healthcare coaching and consulting firm focused on helping clinicians, companies, and medical organizations think clearly under pressure. A practicing urologist and obesity medicine specialist by training, he has spent his career inside the realities this book describes: the clinical demands, administrative burden, professional identity traps, financial pressures, and moral strain that define modern medicine.

Dr. Block's work spans clinical practice, physician coaching, healthcare strategy, biotech and medical device consulting and market adoption analysis. Across those roles, he has advised physicians and healthcare organizations on how systems shape behavior, how professional incentives can quietly distort judgment, and how highly trained clinicians can reclaim agency before burnout becomes collapse.

Burning at Both Ends grew out of that combined perspective: physician, operator, consultant, and colleague. It is written not as an academic treatise or institutional wellness lecture, but as a direct conversation with doctors who still care deeply about medicine but are no longer willing to be consumed by it. Dr. Block's central message is simple: a medical degree is not a life sentence. It is a tool, and it belongs to the physician who earned it.

Also By

Retiring on FIRE: The Fundamental Guide to Retiring Wealthy and Early
The Modern Physician's Survival Guide: How to Grow and Thrive in Modern Healthcare
The Ethical Prince: Power, Realism, and the Art of Leading in a Machiavellian World
Prime After 50: A Urologist's Guide to Strength, Energy, Sex, and Lifelong Vitality

www.ingramcontent.com/pod-product-compliance
Lightning Source LLC
LaVergne TN
LVHW022212200926
848481LV00006B/1943